Voices from the Field
Group Work Responds

Selected Proceedings
Sixteenth Annual Symposium, Association for the Advancement of Social Work with Groups
Hartford, Connecticut
October 27-30, 1994

Executive Board
of the Association for the Advancement
of Social Work with Groups

James Garland, *Chairperson*   Julianne Wayne, *Treasurer*
Maxine Lynn, *Vice-Chairperson*   John Ramey, *General Secretary*
Paul H. Ephross, *Secretary*

Symposium Organizing Committee

Albert S. Alissi   Margaret Darrow   Carolyn Koerner
Joseph Baldwin   Tina Davies   Saul Kutner
Saul Bernstein   Jonathan Foote   Selig Rubinrott
Naomi Blank   Lorrie G. Gardella   Reesa Olins
James Butts   Kasumi Hirayama   Beth Sharkey
Aseh Cole   Edward Hug   Elbert Siegel
Jack Conklin   Mary J. Jean   Justine Stagon
Catherine Cook   Nancy Jessup   Evan Stark
Catherine Corto Mergins   Nancy Klafky   Julianne Wayne
                                                      Raymie Wayne

Special Editors

Tracie Grimley
Edward Hug

Symposium Coordinator

Pamela Wilkie Sakow

HONOREES

Harvey Bertcher   Ivor J. Echols
Ruth Middleman   Daniel Morales

Voices from the Field
Group Work Responds

Albert S. Alissi
Catherine G. Corto Mergins
Editors

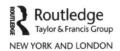

Routledge
Taylor & Francis Group

NEW YORK AND LONDON

First Published by

The Haworth Press, Inc., 10 Alice Street, Binghamton, NY 13904-1580

Transferred to Digital Printing 2010 by Routledge
270 Madison Ave, New York NY 10016
2 Park Square, Milton Park, Abingdon, Oxon, OX14 4RN

Cover design by Marylouise E. Doyle.

Library of Congress Cataloging-in-Publication Data

Voices from the field : group work responds / Albert S. Alissi, Catherine G. Corto Mergins.
    p.   cm.
    Selected proceedings of the 16th annual symposium of the Association for the Advancement of Social Work with Groups.
    Includes bibliographical references and index.
    ISBN 0-7890-0138-1 (alk. paper).
    1. Social group work–Congresses. I. Alissi, Albert S. II. Corto Mergins, Catherine G. III. Association for the Advancement of Social Work with Groups. Symposium (16th : 1994 : Hartford, Conn.)
HV45.V65 1997
361.4–dc21   96-52244
                                                                                                        CIP

Publisher's Note
The publisher has gone to great lengths to ensure the quality of this reprint but points out that some imperfections in the original may be apparent.

CONTENTS

ABOUT THE EDITORS

Albert S. Alissi, DSW, is Professor in the School of Social Work at the University of Connecticut in West Hartford, where he has taught for nearly 30 years. An expert in social group work, group processes, social work and the law, social welfare problems and issues, and multicultural education, he has frequently been called upon as a consultant by organizations such as the Hartford Public Schools, the Connecticut Department of Children and Youth, and the Connecticut Department of Corrections. He is the author of *Perspectives on Social Group Work Practice: A Book of Readings* and *Society and Education in the United States: Racism, Immigration, Deviance.* Professor Alissi's current research interests include self-study methods and the use of action research in social work, pre-release drug treatment recidivism studies, and participant observation studies of homeless men. He is a member of the Academy of Certified Social Workers, the National Association of Social Workers, the Council on Social Work Education, and the American Sociological Association.

Catherine G. Corto Mergins, MSW, is a Social Worker in the Dr. Isaiah Clark Family and Youth Clinic of the Village for Families and Children in Hartford, Connecticut. In this child guidance clinic and school-based setting, she conducts individual and family therapy with children, adolescents, and their families. She also supervises counseling staff in a neighborhood family and youth center. Ms. Corto Mergins has led violence prevention groups for adolescents, Latina mothers' groups focusing on parenting and self-esteem issues, groups for families of homicide victims, and a group for children whose parents have been murdered. A field supervisor for graduate students, she coordinates a summer workshop series for youth employees throughout the city of Hartford. Ms. Corto Mergins is a Licensed Certified Social Worker with the state of Connecticut and is an active member of the National Association of Social Workers and the American Professional Society for the Abuse of Children.

Contributors

John J. Conklin, PhD, Associate Professor, University of Connecticut, School of Social Work, West Hartford, CT.

Kym Crown, CISW, Crown/Gates Associates, West Cronwall, CT.

Kenneth F. Dunker, PhD, Professor of Civil and Constructive Engineering, Iowa State University, Ames, IA.

Hans G. Eriksson, MSW, Director of School for Social Pedagogy, Trondheim, Norway.

Dan Gates, MFT, Crown/Gates Associates, West Cronwall, CT.

J. Jude Gonzales, LSW, Clinical Associate at the University of Illinois Department of Psychiatry, Institute for Juvenile Research, Chicago, IL.

Hisashi Hirayama, DSW, Director, Graduate School of Social Work, University of Tennessee, Memphis, TN.

Kasumi K. Hirayama, DSW, Associate Professor, University of Connecticut, School of Social Work, West Hartford, CT.

Katherine Kohner, MA, Clinical Associate, University of Illinois at Chicago, Institute for Juvenile Research, Chicago, IL.

Gisela Konopka, PhD, Professor Emerita, University of Minnesota, Minneapolis, MN.

Roselle Kurland, PhD, Professor, Hunter College School of Social Work, New York, NY.

Yasuhiro Kuroki, MA, Professor, Doshisha University, Hyoto, Japan.

Judith A. B. Lee, DSW, Professor of Social Work, University of Connecticut, School of Social Work, West Hartford, CT.

Henry W. Maier, PhD, Professor Emeritus at the University of Washington, Seattle, WA.

Flavio Francisco Marsiglia, PhD, Assistant Professor, School of Social Work, Arizona State University, Tempe, AZ.

Mary McKernan McKay, LCSW, PhD, Director of Social Work Training, Clinical Associate, University of Illinois at Chicago, Institute for Juvenile Research, Chicago, IL.

Warren Osterndorf, PhD, Director of Distance Education and Multimedia, Hartford Graduate Center, Hartford, CT.

Mary Lou Paulsen, MSW, Parish Counselor, Bethesda Lutheran Church, IA.

David Ryland, LSW, Clinical Associate at the University of Illinois Department of Psychiatry, Institute for Juvenile Research, Chicago, IL.

Robert Salmon, DSW, Professor, Hunter College School of Social Work, New York, NY.

Susan Stone, LSW, Clinical Associate at the University of Illinois Department of Psychiatry, Institute for Juvenile Research, Chicago, IL.

Joan G. Young, MSW, Director, Hyde Park Center, Family Services of Cincinnati, OH.

Acknowledgments

We are pleased to acknowledge the sponsorship of the University of Connecticut, School of Social Work, the Connecticut Chapter of the Association for the Advancement of Social Work with Groups, and the support of the participating schools of social work–Southern Connecticut State University and St. Joseph College–for their help in making the Symposium a success. We are pleased to acknowledge with gratitude the grants and scholarships provided by The John Martin Foundation, the Northeast Utilities, and the Open Hearth Association.

The editors would also like to pay special tribute to the memories of Norm Goroff and Jim Butts: to Norm, who did so much at the University of Connecticut School of Social Work, in his writings, teachings, and personal face-to-face contacts, to advance the cause of social group work; and to Jim, whose untimely death cut off a most promising teaching career in group work and who spoke so magnificently of the potentials and wonders of cyberspace communications.

And finally, we would like to thank the planning committee, the presenters, session chairpersons, participants, students, and especially the volunteers who worked countless hours, for making it all come together.

Introduction

Albert S. Alissi

Catherine G. Corto Mergins

The Sixteenth Annual Symposium of the Association for the Advancement of Social Work with Groups, Inc., was dedicated to the examination of international contemporary practices of social group workers and the exploration of the potential for enhancing practice knowledge and skills in response to "voices from the field." The program was pursued with two priorities in mind: first, to highlight certain predom-inant themes–comparative group methods, diversity, violence, group care, and education and training that were established as critical areas for the profession in the 1990s; and second, to include as many participants as possible from both the practice and academic fields in the presentations and plenary discussions.

For the second time in its history, the Symposium was held in Hartford, Connecticut, which played host to an impressive gathering of more than 600 participants from around the world. Sessions were varied to accommodate diverse presentations and styles, which included a total of 120 papers, roundtable discussions, workshops, and group members' speak-outs. Pre-symposium institutes were offered, representing a broad spectrum of professional practice and educational themes focusing on theory building, qualitative research, mutual aid, time-limited groups, adventure groups, psychodrama, groups for addictive people and their families, group work with adolescents, administrative groups, private practice, and advanced skill development. The interactive plenaries, invitationals, and special presentations highlighted each of the main symposium themes, which in turn were re-examined in small group sessions. In addition, a media/communication center containing audiovisual equipment and programs featuring group work videos, interactive TV, and a group work computer forum was available to participants throughout the symposium.

The chosen themes inspired all who participated to return to the "roots" of the profession and the work of the "field." Learning from our history, we were challenged to move toward the millennium as visionaries. Gisela Konopka's presentation on "The Meaning of Social Group Work" was a call to renew our commitment to social action through group work and to dedicate not only our profession, but also our lives, to its progress. Henry W. Maier guided us through the historical development of social group work practice and developmental group care and invited us to work toward the continued integration of both in contemporary practice. Judith A. B. Lee brought the empowerment model and the toll of oppression to life with the assistance of shelter staff members, residents, colleagues and life-size puppets. The invitationals provoked us to take a critical look at ourselves as we respond to constantly changing practices in the field.

For four days, clinicians and neighborhood workers, students and professors, researchers and activists, old-timers and newcomers, psychodramatists and adventure therapists, traditionalists and radicals were all held captive by the "power of the group." The air was filled with the electricity of participants conversing, disagreeing, challenging, theorizing, listening, responding, learning, and laughing. Daily newsletter updates kept participants informed of program highlights. A trip to the media center exposed one to the potentials of cyberspace and group work and brought with it the inception of a group work forum on-line. Group work video viewing and taping captured the archives of the profession, as the new developments, interactive learning, and distance education were explored as the latest in teaching technology.

The planning committee's goal to include a diverse range of participants interested in social group work was evidenced in the over 150 multidisciplinary topics that were covered; the number of practitioner grants and student scholarships that were awarded; and the contributions from a significant number of presenters and participants from Canada, Germany, Switzerland, Japan, Australia, and South Africa. It is from these presentations that the following articles have been selected for publication as a representation of the quality, diversity, and challenges presented to the social group work profession in our commitment to social action and personal change. May these pages teach and inspire us as we look toward our future, firmly rooted in our past.

Chapter 1

The Meaning of Social Group Work

Gisela Konopka

It is exciting to see the revival of social group work. Just a few weeks ago, I had a visitor from Hamburg, Germany, who told me how they started to teach it again in departments of education and social work because of its significant philosophy; the period after the Nazis were defeated had brought group work as a most significant part of social work into Germany.

Unfortunately, not enough of this teaching has been brought into the newly developing Russia. Yet, it is most necessary there. In the introduction of a book written in 1994 by American and Russian sociologists, Susan Hartman talks about similarities and differences between Americans and Soviets. One of her sentences struck me: "And although they work in large bureaucracies they have few skills in group interaction and problem-solving" (Maddock, 1994).

In the television program "The Ascent of Man," the scientist Bronowski ended his narration by stepping into a shallow pool of water in the former Auschwitz concentration camp–a pool into which the ashes of thousands of people had been thrown after they were gassed and burned. He scooped up some nearby soil and said, "People must touch each other." James Baldwin wrote about the same idea:

All lives are connected to other lives. Where all human connections are distrusted, the human being is very quickly lost. (Baldwin and Avedon, 1964, p. 84)

We see this loss every day in our work. The problem is not being alone but being isolated, being unconnected, not being counted. It is the vital interrelationship of human beings that is the heart of social group work.

I stuied social group work in 1941, a very short time after I came to this country, after the horrible and demeaning experiences under the Nazis in concentration camps and after living in abject poverty as a refugee in various countries. Having made a decision to fight the Nazis during that time of desperate isolation from the rest of the world and under the constant threat of not just death but torture, one had to decide on the meaning of life. It seemed to me and others that life was useless if one did not stand up for individual dignity and concern for others, regardless of race, national background, or whatever other difference. Yet, translating this basic philosophy into practice was difficult. It required unending courage and complex thinking: Did respect for the individual mean that we should focus only on every single person? Did responsibility for the community mean setting the group ahead of individual concern?

When I first heard about group work I was struck by its exciting promise for a solution to those questions and its capacity for working with people in any field of human endeavor, from community development to education to therapy to work with offenders. Social group work said that the group, the entity that provides a bond among equals, can have the strength to achieve community good and, at the same time, can increase the individuality and creativity of each person within it. And, if necessary, there could be a person, a social group worker, who could help to enhance this freedom and prevent the group from becoming to its members a prison that asks only for conformity. These were exciting insights.

Let me stress again the significant concepts; namely, the equality of members with the group worker (though they don't have the same tasks) and the significance of individuality simultaneous to interdependency. The group worker is a person who is not better than the members, but has, hopefully, a bit more knowledge about, and insight into, group life and functioning. That is, the group worker is not "all-knowing."

About this time 50 years ago, we had to prove to our own profession and to many others that groups could be not only powerful but also helpful. Group work was definitely considered inferior to any one-to-one relationship. Well, we succeeded in convincing people about the significance of groups. But, were we able to clarify what we meant by group work?

I am afraid we were not. We convinced human service professionals of the value of groups, and work with groups has become very fashionable. Yet, the heart of it—the underlying philosophy, the focus on freeing individuals while helping them to support each other—has been lost in an arena of sometimes absurd techniques.

Just a few examples of these techniques will illustrate my point. The mechanistic use of group procedures was brought home to me by a visit to a delinquency institution that is run according to the so-called "scientific" approach of "positive peer culture." The atmosphere in the cottage was a totally inhumane one. Staff was forbidden to develop any positive relationships with the young people, with the rationale that "they must learn to help each other." The adult was only the watchdog. In such an atmosphere, young people learn a language that pretends insight but is only superficial. Their great need for a significant adult who really can listen and respond is overlooked.

Those who cannot stand the kind of pressure brought on by this "technique" become extremely agitated. Adolescents often run away from such treatment. When they are caught, they are adjudicated "delinquent," thus increasing their sense of alienation.

"Confrontation" has become another group work/group therapy game. But confrontation can be helpful only if one knows what he or she is confronting and is not told by someone else who or what one should confront. Also, there is no consideration of the demeaning effect of being yelled at, of being called names, of carrying demeaning signs.

In discussions with adolescents, I found over and over that they felt insulted by group workers and members who constantly "interpreted" and told them what they felt or what they thought. Being in power, we sometimes forget how important self-respect is to other people and especially how fragile it is in children and adolescents.

Consider another example, that of group work based on behavior modification. How can we accept a method and theory whose touchstone is conformity and authoritarianism? One must conform either to the will of the so-called "helper" ("I know what is good for you") or to the group. It lets people learn to behave a certain way only because of consequences imposed on them.

Obedience is demanded in order to achieve discipline within a preson. But this is a discipline that comes from the outside and works only when one is afraid of someone who is stronger than oneself. We do need discipline, an inner discipline, to order our life. What is discipline? To my thinking, it is the opposite of blind obedience. It is the development of a philosophy and a sense of values, a conviction about those values, and the constant effort inside of oneself to put those values into reality, even if this is not comfortable or easy. It does not allow a person an "easy way out"; frequently, it demands that we do the difficult thing. Thomas Etten defined it as an inner discipline that exists when we hold ourselves to what we see as true and real (personal communication).

Adolf Eichmann, on trial for his life because of unspeakable atrocities he committed, said,

> . . . all my life I was used to obedience, since my earliest childhood till May 8, 1945 . . . what profit would disobedience have brought to me, in which way would it have been useful to me? (Eichmann, 1983)

I know that good professionals who base their practice on behavior modification just want to shape behavior with gentle rewards. Certainly all of us do this by encouragement: a hug, a kiss. I have no objection to this. The danger lies in accepting and teaching a false expectation of life.

Not only does behavior modification assume an all-knowing person, it also helps to educate people to expect that life will justly distribute punishment and rewards. The martyrs of all ages, including those of our modern times, such as Ghandi and Martin Luther King, Jr., could testify to the fact that one cannot assume life to be just. Likewise, no reward could be expected by anybody who became actively involved in political action to destroy the Nazis.

In the practice of group work, the rethinking and reaffirmation of a philosophy base are essential. The same applies to community action. Group work's great contribution to community work is its emphasis on self-help, on the strength of ordinary people to accomplish their goals through group association. Mary Follet stressed, "faith in humanity, not faith in poor people or ignorant people, but faith in every living soul" (Konopka, 1958, p. 28). Accordingly, in the practice of group work, there is no condescension and such faith (as described by Follet) helps to break down the concept of "we" and "they." The emphasis on the responsibility of those in need includes the active participation of the people themselves, self-help, and volunteer participation. Social group work speaks of "members," not clients. With this thinking, the practice of social work cannot be restricted to alleviating individual problems, but must also include community action and social reform.

It has always saddened me that in the 1960s our philosophy was not explicit and clear enough, not alive enough in all our practice. As was true for many others in this country, we at times became defensive and were not in the forefront of the beautiful movements of self-assertion, especially of those who thought as well as acted and were not slaves to violent demagogues. I remember that around this time, I became a special assistant to the vice-president of Student Affairs in order to help our university think through the issues of self-government, racial justice, and the translation of dignity of all people into practice through university regulations concerning housing and other aspects of campus life. I was happy to practice social work philosophy, which needs translation into reality wherever there are human beings in turmoil and need. Yet some social workers accused me of having abandoned social work.

It saddened me that it was in this period that schools of social work frequently became very rigid in their admission of students and in the relationship between professors and students, instead of welcoming the beautiful support given by our young people to the basic concept of community in social work. I do know, though, of examples to the contrary as well. I have deep respect for the social workers and social work teachers who did dare to "profess" as times when they were attacked even by their own colleagues. The word "professional" includes "profess." "Profess" means to stand up for one's beliefs, even if it is difficult. I find the dichotomy between direct work and social action totally false. They belong together. In direct practice we experience the excruciating needs—poverty, abuse, being demeaned—and therefore, know the need for change.

When we store the aged in warehouses where they are comparatively well-fed, have a roof over their heads, do not live in filth, but give them no purpose for continued life, this is not fulfilling the need for human dignity. When we do the same with children and young people in institutions where they are regimented to the nth degree, this is not fulfilling human dignity. When we treat colleagues or students with contempt, this is not fulfilling human dignity.

I could go on and name more and far worse instances in which we fulfill basic material needs but violate human dignity. Alan Paton, who himself has been the head of a delinquency institution and who was held prisoner in his own home by a society that would not let him speak up against racial discrimination, said it best:

> To mean something in the world is the deepest hunger of the human soul, deeper than any bodily hunger and thirst, and when a man has lost it, he is no longer a man. (Paton, 1968, p. 19)

And this certainly applies to women as well as men. With the great events in South Africa where finally apartheid is defeated, hope can be regained on the political scene. I wish that in schools of social work in South Africa, social group work will take on one of the major roles.

The translation of social work philosophy into social action is part of practice. Out of the experience of the Nazis, I learned some hard lessons about social action. I want to share the major one, because I see this as part of social group work. Social change cannot be taken for granted. One has to remember that things have to be done over and over again. It is often very hard for me to remember. The task is never finished. The words on the Supreme Court building in Washington, "Eternal vigilance is the price of liberty," surely apply to any effort human beings make.

In the years of Nazi terror, I, as most of us, became very conscious of the fact that one cannot do any significant and positive personal service when the total system does not allow for human dignity. Therefore, political action became far more important than anything else. There were underground movements in Germany that tried to fight an inhumane system that was damaging to young and old. Those who participated could not expect glory, recognition, or even much mutual support. What they could expect was not just death, but painful torture, ridicule, and abandonment.

Dying for a cause is not glamorous as it is so often portrayed in songs, stories, and drama. It is just dying, just not existing anymore. It means mostly being forgotten. We have to remember that there are thousands who did not come out of the Nazi period like me, alive, but did die after very courageously fighting that disastrous system—but nobody will ever talk about them, write about them, or thank them. I resented at that time, and still resent deeply today, those people who shout "social change" and exhort people to action, while they themselves sit in comfortable offices, draw good salaries, gain admiration for what they are doing, but do not face unemployment or persecution as do those whom they exhort to act.

So, I say to myself, do not take the glory if you cannot take the pain. If there is any danger in the way the political action develops, you have to take the risk of this danger. You must have more than the courage of your conviction; you must back it up with your own possessions, or yourself.

For those considerations of group work philosophy, I move into another part of its underlying theory, the understanding of human beings. For too long a time, we imitated the physical sciences, mistook human beings for "things" to be counted, molded, "predicted." Human beings are much too complicated for this. Yet, even the physical sciences, especially physics, have meanwhile learned that they cannot predict all natural events.

Recently I interviewed a 15-year-old in a group home. He told me that it was pretty sad, but since he had been abused as a child, he knows he will abuse others. The absurd theory of predicting human behavior had totally entered his being. It is our task to let people know the strength that is in them and that they can overcome even disastrous experiences.

Also, in working with people, one must never generalize because of a theory. My students often teased me by saying that I have taught them that it was a sin to ever say "the"; for example, "the" adolescent, "the" German, "the" American. We have to understand the uniqueness of every person while we also must understand our commonness. I'd like to quote Thurgood Marshall, who said,

People are people—strike them, and they will cry; cut them, and they will bleed; starve them, and they will wither away and die. But treat them with respect and decency, give them equal access to the levers of power, attend to their aspirations and grievances, and they will flourish and grow and . . . join together to "form a more perfect union."

To continue making contributions to the great promise of social group work, we must continue to develop a philosophy of *freedom with boundaries and understanding of human beings in interaction with others and their environment* as a basis for competent practice.

To do this, we need scholar-practitioners, not timid bureaucrats or status-seeking individuals. We need–and I know we have among us–people "with winged feet and burning hearts" to whom "nothing human is alien." We need compassion. I am ending with a poem written by a young man in a group home and given to me by him:

Looking into the shattered mirror, you'll see the pain of a lost child.
The child lost to a world of Hell:
Look deeper into the mirror. You'll see the sadness of the child, the pain, the hurt.
Don't look, you'll be sorry. It's something so painful your eyes will hurt and tears will burn down your face.
Why, you'll ask, has this child had to live this life?
The broken child, the shattered life. Look, you'll know how deep the hatred is. Look in the mirror.
Look in my eyes, the mirror of the soul.

To work with such pain we must reaffirm group work's demand and promise: significance of the individual, mutual help, and equality between the helper and those who need help. It is not easy, but it can be done.

REFERENCES

Baldwin, James and Avedon, Richard. (1964). *Nothing Personal*, NY: Atheneum.

Eichmann, Adolf. (1983). *Eichman Interrogates: Transcripts from the Achieves of the Israel Police*. J. Von Lang (Ed.). New York: Farrar, Straus & Giroux.

Konopka, Gisella. (1958). *Eduard C. Lindeman and Social Work Philosophy*, Minneapolis: University Press.

Maddock, James W. (1994). *Families Before and After Perestroika*. New York: Guilford Press.

Patton, Alan (1968). *Long View*. E. Callan (Ed.). New York: F.A. Praeger.

Chapter 2

Social Group Work and Developmental Group Care: Retrospect and Prospects for Both

Henry W. Maier

This chapter deals with out-of-home care where the practice of both social group work and developmental group care can have a vital part in the service agenda. I trust that my major emphasis on contemporary issues will enhance the challenge for the integration of both of these practice approaches, which have considerable commonality.

First, let me define developmental group care and social group work as I see it. Developmental group care practice, sometimes called "milieu-based group work" (Garland, 1994, p. 159), entails the *interactions*, individually or as a group, between group care workers and children, youth, or adults, who are temporarily apart from their families. Thus, in developmental group care, workers strive for *primary* relationship experience. Care work is consequently oriented to the utilization of daily life events for therapeutic purposes and *is* the essence of effective care practice. This focus on the ordinary daily life experience distinguishes this practice from other helping approaches in the human relations field.

In contrast, social group work practice addresses personal and social issues of members who live essentially in an open society and who, overall, have continuous linkages with their families and neighborhood.

One more clarification might be in order. The usual terms of "caretaking" and "caregiving" I purposely have replaced with "*interactional care*," because "caregiving" or "care taking" tend to imply a *one*-directional, hierarchical-prone process. Actually, these processes entail a *reciprocal exchange*. The use of the term *care interactions* highlights the mutuality of the exchange; moreover, the giving and receiving can occur for both parties. Care practitioners are apt to experience a sense of being personally worthwhile while also gaining a degree of professional competence assurance. I contend that there is growth, although different for each one involved. (It is interesting to note that Larry Shulman [1993] implies that a similar notion of interactional approach is also applicable to social *group work.*)

IN RETROSPECT

In retrospect, social group work has offered limited but remarkable input to group care introduced by social group workers. Just to note a few, there is the pioneering work of Fritz Redl and Dave Wineman (1957); Gisela Konopka (1965, 1970); Mary Lee Nicholson (1975, 1979); Alex Gitterman (1984); Edith Moore (1978) Edith Moore and Audrey J Starkes (1992); Toby Berman-Rossi (1986); Tom Douglas (1986); and I am sure that there are many others in the front lines of practice who have not yet found recognition in the literature.

In my reflections on the past I realized with pleasure that social group workers have long led groups across the age span. They pursued original and untraditional work with elders and also persons in transition, on the streets, in waiting rooms, in shelters, or on the waysides (e.g., Holmes-Garrett, 1984). Additionally, it seems that we have heard Florence Ray Stier's admonishment that group work as a treatment method should not be merely "patched onto the institutional programs by hiring a [social] group worker" (Ray, 1965, p. 6). Furthermore, it is true that group workers have lent their efforts to mental health and medical care settings but apparently were less visible in child welfare, correctional, and penal institutional systems.

In 1954, a child- and youth-care training program, spawned within the Psychiatric and Child Development Department of the University of Pittsburgh, was turned down in its request to become a part of the University's School of Social Work. Group *care* practice was then not conceived within their sphere of interest. Today, forty years later, the group care educational sequence is a fully accepted, enriching and enriched part and parcel of that school. *Change is possible!* Similarly, at a major mid-western university, its school of social work has currently approached the independent child and youth care work division in order to link up with them for joint educational endeavors.

In the past, social group workers in residential settings dealt with individual treatment adaptation, including mediational issues between group members and the organization. At the same time, group workers tended to hold on to their professional identity, striving to remain free of bureaucratic alignments. Altogether, in retrospect, social group workers established small but valid efforts in the group care field.

PROSPECTS: HUMAN GROWTH
AND DEVELOPMENTAL REQUIREMENTS

The present and near future of social group work and developmental group care practice I see as exciting for the possibility of mutual acknowledgement and enrichment of each. Both forms of practice will need future progress to advance their attention to developmental human growth experience. Group members are not merely in groups to find mutual support, social enhancement, and possibly rehabilitation within the context of peers and worker. They also need all along the life span to grow and develop. Human beings' natural life development is as much at stake as any problem-solving requirements within group care, as well as in social group work practice (Shulman, 1993; Garland, 1994; Maier, 1991). Group care can also learn but *not* copy practice approaches from our European friends, the Educateurs (Garland, 1994). (Let me add quickly that imports from Europe are not necessarily bad!)

In connection with the foregoing recommendations, we might remind ourselves of the conceptual difference between "associate groups" and those that have "primary care" as a major objective. In associate groups (1), that is, in social group work traditionally members and worker join together for specific interests or problems about personal or external demands. At the same time, they see themselves and *are* seen as part of their respective ongoing primary family and community networks. On the other hand, group care has historically focused upon primary care; that is, to be engaged with individuals who must live apart from and often are completely cut off from their original primary contacts (family, neighborhood peers, and their community) (Maier, 1978, p. 203). Essentially, these are the persons in group care programs. Group care stands for them as a potential resource for the development of temporary *primary life connections*, a bridge for establishing or re-establishing permanent relationships (Maier, 1991; 1994).

Consequently, group care practice envisages the objective that every person, young or old, regardless of social circumstances, requires that there is a sound alignment with at least one care person (Bronfenbrenner, 1979; Maier, 1994). Ultimately, joint living and continuous, healthy close attachment with one or the other care person will hopefully provide connections leading to greater self-control and the ability to proceed independently on one's own in the absence of the attached worker. Eventually, attachment will strengthen the ability to proceed on one's own. In short, *attachment frees* (Maier, 1987, Chapter 5).

Attention to developmental growth, especially to attachment nurturance, seems to become increasingly essential within the current North American practice scenes where so many children, youth, and older adults appear to drift on their own or find themselves in a void with a dearth of roots and personally enriching connections (Anderson, 1994). For them, nurturance of primary developmental processes becomes particularly significant. They need genuine *human* connections far beyond problem-solving efforts. They require personal nurturing attachment experience over time in order that they can discover that they *are* somebody and that they are worthy partners in our diverse society (Anderson 1994; Shulman, 1993).

Such a powerful reminder challenges us to become more aware of today's urgent necessity for *life care* groups in the streets, shelters, and prisons, along with the ones in group care settings. The creation of *life care* ventures is not a mere rescue operation; it represents society's acknowledgment of its partnership in human development. We learned from our native forebears that it takes a village to raise a child. We are now catching up with the recognition that societal involvement is absolutely essential all along the life course (VanderVen, 1992; Maier, 1992). These kinds of connections are neither a last resort nor a remedial aid; it is self-evident that when family, school, and other primary contacts seem to lose their influence, primary group care affiliations are in natural demand. Group experience can assist with such life decision-making processes (Shulman, 1993) to provide recognition of the value of the human being, with guidance for personal hygiene and for sexual behaviors, with making friends in a diversified neighborhood, and with other vital personal boundary issues (Anderson, 1994). Most likely, group workers' current attention to routine life skills training has to be expanded to include these personal life-oriented tasks.

Additionally, social group work with its decisive commitment to values for *participatory interactions, mutual aid, and for a strong reliance upon membership power* (Nadelman, 1986, p. 143; Moore and Starkes, 1992, pp. 185-186) can enrich group care practice where an almost self-appointed zeal suggests that workers themselves have to do it all on their own (Moore and Starkes, 1992).

ISSUES FOR THE INTERFACE
OF SOCIAL GROUP WORK
AND DEVELOPMENTAL GROUP CARE

As an interface challenge, social group work and developmental group care, as partners of the social sciences, are absorbing powerful paradigm changes. First, there is alteration from an intra-psychic view to one with an *interactional* perspective. Secondly, human relation efforts are asked to find ways for incorporating *contextual* factors as part of their holistic work scene (Bronfenbrenner, 1979; Moore, 1983, pp. 27-29; Moore and Starkes, 1992, p. 182). These widening perspectives give developmental group care an added shove to assume an open systems stance, utilizing small face-to-face groups amid the network of structured organization-oriented groups (Bronfenbrenner, 1979). Such an ecological approach verifies systems thinking and negates for alternate group practices the erroneous assumption of groups as independent and freestanding.

Additionally, both group care and group work approaches have to give attention to the pitfalls of small group practices. An example would be the institutional exploitation of peer pressures and the inherent pull toward conformity (Resnick, 1980) in contrast to parochial peer values where peer attachment and loyalty are utilized to carry out the expectation of adult standards. Moreover, if we strive to have individuals able to say "no" on the street, they probably need first to learn it "on location" in their living groups. Social group workers can here lend experience, knowledge, and value-orientation (Nadelman, 1986).

Finally, in the interface of both practices, social group workers are confronted by a demand that the continuum of work be expanded to a process of individual follow-up with former group members and their families or other significant contacts. Follow-up work also points, nowadays, to attending to research in regard to the efficacy of change efforts in their respective groups (Guterman et al., 1989).

CHILDREN BE CHILDREN, YOUTH BE YOUTHFUL, AND ADULTS ALLOW THEMSELVES TO BE PLAYFUL

One of the major dilemmas and challenges of our times seems to be to let children be *children*, youth to be *youthful*, and to grant adults permission to be *joyfully playful*, each in their respective ways. It seems that major trends in contemporary thinking, including in our own professional ambitions, have difficulties in granting permission to the young to be *young* and to older ones to be still young at heart. This has applications for the workers and social services while they deal with the fierce complexities with which people are faced as they require our services. In fact, it might be true for the workers themselves. Ruby Pernell (1991) wondered at an earlier Annual Meeting whether *spontaneity* is still highly valued in our social group work.

It seems that there is presently very little room left for light-hearted and frivolous behaviors in the group care fields. Token economy, level programs, and the strong value placed upon maintenance work leave so little space for finding healthier ways of living. Moreover, I wonder whether group care has become in some instances a place for janitorial training. It is so easy to forget, especially in the children and youth care fields, that these youngsters may have to be helped first to be *children*. Practitioners, administrators, and policy makers need to support each other to foster human beings' inherent spontaneous potentials! Along these lines, group workers can help group care in finding more activities for potential enjoyment and modes of interactions. There is an urgent need for stimulating activities geared at an age level *below* that of the youngsters in care. Workers sometimes feel inhibited to encourage exuberant play, especially if these activities promise or threaten to lead to loud noise or momentary breakdown of expendable controls. Group work has much to offer with its rich history in programming and a healthy disposition toward enjoyment of life (Barnes, 1991, p. 135). Such an orientation is urgently opportune in the face of these production-oriented days, where there is a need to validate the importance of idle times and good, sound loafing. I think there is a need for a fifth basic freedom: *A FREEDOM TO RELAX and BE JOYFUL!*

FAMILY PRESERVATION

Family preservation efforts, a contemporary vogue and a valuable necessity, focus upon enhancing family connections at all times. Family preservation is geared toward linking together estranged or splintered members and especially maintaining children and youth within their own families (Whittaker, 1978). For group work practice, persons' severe level of stress coupled with the absence of family ties have become presently an urgent concern for social intervention. This is a value-imperative that has real implications for group work practitioners (Ainsworth and Fulcher, 1994).

For group care practice, it has already made a difference. It is important, however, to address the fact that some of the major tasks of family preservation work fall upon the shoulders of the care workers, the ones who receive the least training and recognition, while they have to carry the major load and strain of the group care effort. They are now expected to be at hand when the youngsters and their respective family members come together. After all, if personal contacts are to flourish, much has to happen after they have exchanged their *initial "hello."* Here, group work has widely accumulated experience for such potentially conflict-laden encounters. Care workers have much to learn in order to prepare the individuals and their family members prior to these reunions. Most importantly, there is the *how, where, when,* in particular *what to do,* and *which immediate supports should be at hand.* Group work and group care might open up new venues for their joint learning toward enriched modes of services. There is, for example, the rich accumulated experience of group work with "beginnings" and beyond, as well as multi-generational groups (Barth, 1994; Hearn, 1991).

NEW TIMES, NEW AVENUES OF SERVICE

In these changing times, new paradigms replace previous ones. Lateral or latest know-how and peer orientation outdate hierarchical and traditional stances (Maier, 1974). There is an awakening attention to *inter*dependence in lieu of the high value once placed on "independence," with its associated aversion to dependence. It seems *interdependence* is the preferred mode for the days to come. Consequently, the fostering of *interdependent experiences* with consequent mutual growth predictively is the lot for workers and other group members in our fields. The latter entails ultimate commitment and skills in participatory group care practice as we recognize the potential for change via small group interaction. Another important emphasis is group care's experience with growth-oriented delivery of services for all ages. I see a challenge for all of us to forge ahead, working no longer parallel but closely together. With the changes of *what* to do, adjustments will occur about *who* will do it.

In another area, human services are called upon to relate to processes of *transitions* in primary relationship alignments (Krueger, 1994), *transitions* in secondary and community commitments, and, always, *transitions* throughout the progression of the life span (VanderVen, 1992). These are all features within the province of group care and group work. Group work practice may have to include additional knowledge with regard to *developmental care,* especially pertaining to adult development. On the other hand, planners for group care may have to acquire some of group work's ready support for groups' internal and external thrust toward empowerment.

In the preceding paragraphs, thus far I trust it has become apparent that social group work and developmental group care have one basic perspective in common. In neither form of practice is a major emphasis put upon worker input, nor upon structured activities, nor do they build upon group members' insight or behavioral learning. They do, however, focus upon the EXPERIENCE, which all parties involved have *together with each other.* The nature of the minutae of every respective joint experience defines what actually has impacted each person. (For group work see Shulman, 1993; for group care see Maier, 1991.) This commonality is not only striking, it is unifying (Moore and Starkes, 1992, p. 184). James Garland recently observed, "Social group work is so remarkably together with milieu child and youth care purpose and approaches" (1994, p. 159).

In closing, it might be relevant to echo Gisela Konopka's reminder. Members of "the helping professions must continue to speak up for a service that needs to be improved" (1965, p. 25). And I can probably best sum up my observations with Garland's pointed reminder: Let's talk about what we social workers and milieu-based group workers can *do* together. *"If not us, who will do what needs to be done for our children"* and other age groups (1994, p. 160).

REFERENCES

Ainsworth, F. and L. Fulcher. (1994). The function of recent service development in child welfare. Boston: (Manuscript for publication).

Anderson, E. (1994). The code of the street. *Atlantic Monthly.* March: 81-94.

Barnes, H.F. (1991). From warehouse to greenhouse: Play, work and the routines of daily living in groups as the core of milieu treatment. In Beker, J. and Z. Eisikovits. (Eds.). *Knowledge Utilization: Residential Child & Youth Care Practice.* Washington, DC: Child Welfare League of America. pp. 123-155.

Barth, R.P. (1994). Shared family care: Child protection and family preservation. *Social Work.* 39(5): 515-524.

Berman-Rossi, T. (1986). The fight against hopelessness institutionalized aged. In Gitterman, A. and L. Shulman. *Mutual Aid Groups and the Life Cycle.* Itasca, IL: F.R. Peacock, Publisher. pp. 33-357.

Bronfenbrenner, U. (1979). *The Ecology of Human Development.* Cambridge, MA: Harvard University Press.

Douglas, T. (1986). *Group Living.* London: Tavistock Publication. Especially pp. 166-197.

Garland, J.A. (1994). An editorial. *Child & Youth Care Forum.* 23(3), 159-160.

Gitterman, A. (1984). Building supports in groups. *Social Work with Groups.* 12(2): 5-21.

Guterman, N.B., V.G. Hodges, B.J. Blythe, and R.L. Brown (1989). Aftercare service development for children in residential treatment. *Child & Youth Care Quarterly.* 18(2): 119-130.

Hearn, B. (1991). *Settings of Family Group Projects.* London: Longman.

Holmes-Garrett, C. (1984). The crisis of the forgotten: A single session in the ICU waiting room. *Social Work with Groups.* 12(4): 141-157.

Konopka, G. (1965). Group work in residential treatment: A historical review. In H.W. Maier (Ed.). *Group Work As Part of Residential Treatment.* New York: National Association of Social Work. pp. 13-25.

———— (1970). *Group Work in the Institution.* New York: The Association Press.

Krueger, M.A. (1994). *In Transition.* Milwaukee, WI. (Manuscript for publication.)

Maier, H.W. (1974). A sideward look at change and what comes into view. In *Social Work In Transition.* Seattle, WA School of Social Work, University of Washington Publication. pp. 138-147.

———— (1978). *Three Theories of Child Development: Piaget, Erikson, and Sears.* New York: Harper & Row, Publishers (Third Edition).

———— (1987). *Developmental Group Care of Children And Youth: Theory and Practice.* Binghamton, NY: The Haworth Press.

———— (1991). An exploration of the substance of child and youth care practice. *Child & Youth Care Forum.* 20(6): 393-411.

———— (1992). The substance of care practice throughout the life span. *Journal of Child & Youth Care.* 7(4): 79-91.

———— (1994). Attachment development is "in." *Journal of Child & Youth Care.* 9(1): 35-51.

Moore, E.E. (1978). The implications of system networks for social work. *Social Work with Groups.* 3(2), 133-143.

———— (1983). The group-in-situation as the unit of attention in social work with groups. *Social Work with Groups.* 6(2): 19-31.

Moore, E.E. and A.J. Starkes (1992). The group-in-institution as the unit of attention: Recapturing and refining a social work tradition. *Social Work with Groups.* 15(2/3): 171-192.

Nadelman, A. (1986). Sharing the hurt: Adolescents in a residential setting. In A. Gitterman and L. Shulman. *Mutual Aid Groups: The Life Cycle.* Itasca, IL: F.E. Peacock, Publishers. pp. 141-159.

Nicholson, M.L. (1975). Child care practice and the passion of today: Some propositions. *Child Care Quarterly.* 4(2): 72-83.

———— (1979). Fateful moments when one abides children to enter time. Gisela Konopka Lecture.

Pernell, R. (1991). Mis-use, non-use, under-use, maxi-use (in another five years) of a social work method. In Weil, K., K. Chan and D. Southerland (Eds.) *Theory and Practice In Social Group Work.* Binghamton, NY: The Haworth Press. pp. 39-51.

Ray, F. (1965). Foreword. In Maier, H.W. (ed.). *Group Work As Part of Residential Treatment.* New York: The National Association of Social Work. pp. 5-7.

Redl, F. and D. Wineman. (1957). *The Aggressive Child.* New York: Basic Books, Inc.

Resnick, H. (1980). A social system view of strain. In Resnick, H. and R. Patti. *Change from Within.* Philadelphia, PA: Temple University Press. pp. 28-45.

Shulman, L. (1993). Developing and testing a practice theory: An interactional perspective. *Social Work.* 38(1): 91-97.

VanderVen, K. (Ed.). (1992). Care practice throughout the life span. *Journal of Child & Youth Care.* 7(4). (The entire issue is devoted to this topic.)

Whittaker, J.K. (1978). The changing character of residential child care: An ecological perspective. *Social Service Review.* 52(1): 21-36.

Chapter 3

The Empowerment Group in Action: My Sisters' Place

Judith A. B. Lee with My Sister's
Place group members
and Ruth R. Martin

INTRODUCTION

I have been asked to "recapture" this presentation for the Proceedings. This is not easy, as it became quite a moving happening
for all present. It included a brief talk defining the empowerment
group approach, a sociopolitical drama (a code), and two empowerment group meetings–a meeting within a meeting, as it were. The
My Sister's Place (MSP) group presented their own reflections on
the code/dramatic enactment, and the group and the audience entered into dialogue creating a live empowerment group.

I decided to present in this way, to include the audience in an
actual empowerment group experience, rather than just make a
speech on empowerment groups. I thank Al Alissi and Catherine
Corto Mergins, co-chairs, for making this experience possible. Having the Symposium in Hartford gave me a unique opportunity to
involve the women and staff of My Sisters' Place (MSP) in presenting their work in their own voices rather than just referring to them
as silent "co-authors" of the empowerment approach. MSP is a

The MSP empowerment group members were Judith Beaumont, Rosalind
Moore-Beckham, Gail Bourdon, Jean Konon, Stacey Miles, and Christy King;
children, Marley and Channel Maxwell; and Ruth R. Martin, Invited Griot/Elder.

three-program (and growing) agency serving homeless and former-ly homeless women and children in inner-city Hartford.

The practice experiences that most influenced my conceptualiza-tion of the empowerment approach and the development of the empowerment group concept were my work in a New York City shelter for homeless women (Lee, 1991, 1992; 1994a*,b) and my work at My Sisters' Place in Hartford, Connecticut (Lee, 1991; 1994a). These experiences involved consultation and direct prac-tice. The dialogue and political activism with administration, staff, and group members prompted my own reflections on oppression, and its practice across race, class, and many other lines, and em-powerment. The work at MSP also provided a very special support and empowerment group for me. How wonderful it would be, I thought, for my dear group work colleagues, whose work upon which I have built, to share a group meeting with me. How good it would be if my MSP colleagues and my group work colleagues could dialogue with each other on the oppressions we all experience in a society where 1 percent of the population controls 37 percent of the wealth and the top 10 percent of extremely rich white men control 86 percent of the wealth (West, 1993).

With this goal of empowering dialogue in mind, I asked two members of the Successful Women's Group (Lee, 1994a) and the executive director and program directors of MSP (who also practice directly with empowerment groups) to join me in an empowerment group "happening," which we would present at the Symposium as a vehicle for dialogue. This group was the blending of an MSP "client" group and staff group. I had worked with each separately at MSP, and it was only a small leap to put both of these groups together. We also included two children who had participated in political demonstrations while living at MSP and wanted to be part of the dramatic enactment/code. We decided to add one last person to complete this intergenerational group, our colleague and friend, Dr. Ruth R. Martin, African-American oral history scholar (1994) and associate dean at the University of Connecticut School of So-

---

*This chapter contains some paraphrases from *The Empowerment Approach to Practice* by Dr. Judith A. B. Lee. (Copyright © 1994 by Columbia University Press. Reprinted with permission of the publisher.)

cial Work. We invited Ruth to have a special, culturally appropriate, group member's role: that of African-American elder/griot/story-teller. In that role, she would bring words of encouragement to our reconstituted empowerment group by bringing the wisdom of the past to the present struggle. Empowerment work is difficult as it demands both personal and political raising of consciousness. Enacting it before a large group is even more difficult. Ruth's role of giving to this group of black and white members out of her experience would add to our strength in this process. She would be the "indigenous" group leader, and I would be the worker for the group. Now that I have introduced the group members, I will follow the format of the presentation.

THE EMPOWERMENT APPROACH AND THE EMPOWERMENT GROUP

The empowerment group is a particular type of group that grows out of and embodies the principles, values, theoretical foundations, methodology, and skills of the empowerment approach to social work practice (Lee, 1994a). The empowerment approach is not value neutral. As Gisela Konopka noted, groups are not good per se, they can be used for good or evil (Knopka, 1988). Ruby Pernell emphasized, in her keynote speech at the Sixth Annual AASWG Symposium, that by definition empowerment is political and contains the intention to change the status quo (1986). The value base of the empowerment approach includes a preferential option to work alongside people who are poor and who have experienced oppression for a variety of reasons. There are eight principles, which include "people empower themselves," as well as self-empowerment "should be assisted by the social worker" but "people need each other" to raise consciousness and act to relieve the conditions of oppression that may be externally imposed and internally incorporated. Hence the empowerment approach is both personal/clinical and political. It is a both/and conceptualization.

The empowerment approach specifically addresses social work practice with people who experience blocks (internalized and external) to attaining the resources needed to enjoy the fullness of life by virtue of stigmatized collective identities (Solomon, 1976). Class, race, gender, and difference (related to physical or mental challenge, age, religion, sexual orientation, etc.) are strong predictors of experiencing oppression. It may take the form of prejudice, stereotypes, discrimination, and blocked opportunity systems and life chances. The empowerment approach blends the personal/sometimes clinical and political/structural levels of the changes needed to transform and liberate people who experience oppression.

The "live example" of a staff and client group addressing issues of homelessness in an affluent America exemplifies and is a prototype of the empowerment approach. The approach can be utilized in the one-to-one, small-group, community, or political arena. The small group is the critical unit in most of these constellations. The key processes are dialogue and praxis: action-reflection and action in a circular loop, which includes consciousness-raising and transformation. Such activities as building pride in peoplehood and community and analyzing on the personal, systemic, and wider societal levels are integral parts of the approach. Building on strengths and taking personal responsibility for change are also key concepts. Women who are homeless, for example, may also need to address issues of self-esteem, competence/skills, relatedness, self-direction/autonomy, and identity even as they seek to change their own situations and address the lack of affordable housing. The support, caring, and mutual aid of peers is essential in this difficult process.

WHAT IS EMPOWERING IN EMPOWERMENT GROUPS?

Most groups have empowering qualities in that they provide different perspectives on common struggles as well as an opportunity for mutual aid, caring, community, and collective action. In the empowerment group the common struggles *explicitly* include issues of oppression. So, for example, empowerment groups at MSP focus on various facets of homelessness and personal and political actions to end it. They go beyond the solution of rehousing individual members to making systemic changes locally (and beyond) in the programs and policies that contribute to the problem. Additionally, they openly address issues of racism, sexism, classism, and other "isms" in everyday life. Ultimately, they aim toward restructuring views of self-efficacy, in a society that says some people are more worthwhile than others, and political action. They make connections between personal pain and societal structures.

Blending a critical education method (Freire, 1973) with an inter-actionist/mutual aid and mainstream group approach (Schwartz, 1974; Papell and Rothman, 1980) the empowerment group becomes its own unique group type. The posing of questions about societal structures and inequities and, hence, the raising of consciousness is equally important to finding solutions to immediate concerns through group process.

To be empowering, the group itself must attain power to the extent its composition, time span, and structure permit. The groups in the shelter are open-ended. As composition changes, the power of the group to fulfill its purposes and develop as a group vacillates. Some groups develop an ongoing nucleus over several months, and these groups do attain this power. Others last only a week or so and have much less power. In the transitional living facility for women and families and in the scattered site housing programs for persons with mental illness, groups exist over long periods of time with relatively stable composition and can become powerful.

I will now discuss some ways to help empowerment groups empower themselves as groups.

Promote Groupness

According to Wood and Middleman (1989), to promote "groupness" the worker begins by helping the group members gain a sense of each other and their groupness. She encourages the development of a mutual aid system by promoting member-to-member communication. Next, the worker respects and utilizes group process as the central change dynamic. Then, the worker works to do herself out of a job, helping the group increase its autonomy. The practitioner needs to be able to "think group"; that is to understand group structure and dynamics and to utilize group focused skills in working with groups. Social work practice with groups must appreciate and utilize the group as a whole as the helping system. In empowerment groups, the worker must "think empowerment" in process and outcomes as well.

Use Free-Form Communication

Wood and Middleman (1989) distinguish types of communication in groups, which may affect the development of the group as a mutual aid system: "The Maypole," where the worker talks to individuals one-by-one and dominates and controls the group; "The Round Robin," where each participant speaks in turn in relation to a given focus by a worker who is still in control; "The Hot Seat," where the worker maintains control and engages in an extended conversation with a member while the others are an audience; "The Agenda Controlled" group, where new and old business and Robert's Rules dominate; and, finally, "The Free Form," where participants take responsibility to speak with any other person according to the dictates of the moment. Here, the primary responsibility for the flow and form of the work rests with the participants who observe matters of turn-taking, consideration, and risking. This latter form of communication is the optimal pattern for empowering groups.

Relinquish the Role of Expert

Norma Lang (1986) notes that the worker must relinquish the role of expert as clinician or teacher and promote member-to-member transactions. This does not mean that the worker withholds his or her knowledge or expertise but that he or she shares it without taking center stage, recognizing that members are experts in their own realities. The worker must maximize the group members' potential for helping each other and for taking over their own leadership and direction.

Utilize a Mixed Goals Group Form

Many practitioners preserve the dyadic relationship in the group through one-on-one communication patterns. Lang identifies four group form. The first is *the individual goals group*, where influence flows unilaterally from the worker or the group members to each individual and toward individual goal accomplishment. In this form, the group itself may not be fully developed. The *collective goals group* employs the fully developed group toward the realization of collectively held goals. In *the shared goals group*, there is a strong reciprocal influence capable of meeting the needs of its members. Finally, in *the mixed goals group*, some combination of these goals operates together in a multiple goals context with some sequencing of goals. In such groups the source of influence is compounded, coming from both group and worker. Individual and collective empowerment goals may, therefore, be met.

The empowering group includes provisions for meeting individual needs through group processes and can best be described as a mixed goals group form in which a freeform style of communication is used. Group methods, techniques, and skills, which develop the group's power while attending to the needs of individual members, are empowering in both process and outcomes.

In addition to building on the mutual aid group type, which ideally utilizes the empowering mechanisms named above, the empowerment group builds on critical education principles.

CRITICAL EDUCATION
AND CONSCIENTIZATION

Alienated people, particularly poor people, often develop a culture of passive silence and apathy about their situations. For the poor of Brazil, the problem of developing awareness was compounded by illiteracy. Paulo Freire (1973) used critical education to develop literacy and to develop critical thinkers who could transform their own societies.

Critical education means to confront, reflect on, and evaluate the problems and contradictions of society in order to change them. Critical awareness develops in a process of dialogue with others in groups. The development of critical awareness is called *conscientization* (Freire, 1973). The basic elements of Freire's method included the following:

• Participant observation of educators/workers who "tune-in" to the vocabular universe of people
• An arduous search for words (and themes) rich in experiential involvement

- A codification of these words into visual images—pictures, charts, and skits—which stimulate people submerged in the culture of silence to emerge as conscious makers of their own culture
- The decodification by the culture circle and coordinator/worker in dialogue
- A creative new codification explicitly critical and aimed at action

The roles of the coordinator/worker are to problematize the situation; to pose critical questions about reality that group participants experience; and to codify, decodify, reflect on, act on, reflect again (praxis), and develop their own awareness (Freire, 1973).

This critical education method has many parallels to social work with empowerment groups. Pence (1987) and others have used Freire's critical education method in working with battered women. She suggests that the group (1) begin with a survey of what is on people's minds; (2) choose a theme, posing problems in question form; (3) analyze the problems on the personal, institutional (systems), and cultural levels; (4) develop a code (picture, chart, play, poem) that stimulates thinking and feeling to further reflect on the problem; and (5) develop options for action in all three areas of analysis, then act together and reflect again. (See Lee, 1994a, especially Figure 8.1, p. 223-224.) Today we are illustrating the use of a code to stimulate reflection on homelessness and women and children of color. We hope action will not lag far behind. The code is in the form of a sociopolitical drama.

THE EMPOWERMENT GROUP

In summation, the empowerment group utilizes the principles, knowledge base, and skills of the empowerment approach and explicitly defines empowerment as purpose, content, process, and outcome of the group's work (Lee, 1994a). It is not a support or mutual-aid group, nor a "therapeutic group," nor is it a consciousness-raising or critical education group, nor a political action group. It is all of the above and, by its unique combination of these, more.

Empowerment groups are appropriate for persons who face issues of pervasive external and internalized oppression in their lives. Children and youth as well as adults and elders may benefit from empowerment groups. By definition, such groups contain social action and social change goals as well as personal and interpersonal ones. These broad purposes are offered to group members who then determine what external power blocks, deficits, or shortages and areas of internalized oppression and other personal problems need to be addressed, and how they want to address them. Sometimes people who experience pervasive oppression are so accustomed to living with it that they assume "that's just the way things are." An initial consciousness-raising effort is then needed in order to include oppression in the problem definition. To attain empowerment, one has to name one's power problems and locate them in personal struggles and in the fabric of a society that seeks to marginate persons of difference. Then group members must work to change the power balance in their favor. The worker may initially need to name experiences of oppression for what they are, but will soon find that those who suffer are well able to develop the themes as they pursue empowerment.

THE CODE/SOCIOPOLITICAL DRAMA

In this and the final two sections, I will reconstruct a somewhat modified process recording of the code and the empowerment group meeting that took place. (See also Mistry, 1995.)

As the "graduates"/Successful Women and staff of MSP and Dr. Martin take their places in the rear of the room with the greater-than-life-size puppets, I invite the members of the audience to become part of the group in experiencing and decoding the code the women have constructed to take us deeper into the dynamics of oppression and homelessness. I ask all present to enter into the drama affectively, and then we will decode it together on the personal, institutional/systemic, and cultural/societal levels.

Dr. Ruth Martin leads the procession dressed in African garb and beating a slow rhythm on the drum. Following is Channel Maxwell, age 9, who is distributing large "dollar bills" to the audience. On the reverse side, they state how much of the American tax dollar goes to militarism and how much to social services, including affordable housing ("less than 2 cents on the dollar"). Then a huge "Uncle Sam" puppet with a skeletal face and hands looms over us.

Judy Beaumont carries the body as Jean Konon and Rosalind Moore-Beckham ominously wave each arm over the crowd. Marley Maxwell, a small but sturdy Afro-Caribbean 13-year-old, follows dragging a large wooden cross over his shoulder. He stumbles and rights himself. A black-shrouded woman of color puppet brings up the rear. Beneath the black robe, Gail Bourdon tips the tearful face with her mouth fixed in a silent cry of pain toward those nearest. Christy King and Stacey Miles move each arm to cover her face, to plead for mercy, to beg for help, to share her grief. The procession slowly winds to the left and the right of the room, finally assembling before the group.

As this happens, I share 1989 statistics regarding poverty and infant and child mortality in the United States. I ask "why" in relation to each statement. For example, why is the poverty line set so low? Seventeen percent of all American children live in poverty with almost 10 percent (9.8%) living below the horrendously low poverty line of $12,500 for a family of four. The poverty rate for black and Hispanic children now approaches 50 percent. The United States is tied with Singapore and New Zealand as nineteenth in global ratings of infant

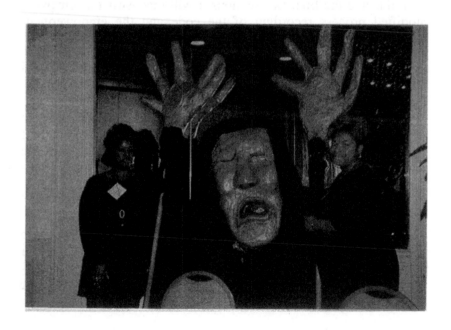

and child mortality. Children, then the aged, are the poorest groups in the United States. The numbers of children are dramatically increasing in the almost three million people found homeless on any given night in the United States. To avoid homelessness one needs a six-month reserve of income. Ruth beats the drum quickly several times, then stops. The procession faces the audience. Marley puts his arms over each side of the cross and bows his head. The Mourning Mother throws her arms into the air. Uncle Sam turns his back.

The drama is over.

The Group Meeting

There is silence. Some members of the group/cast and audience members exhale heavily as the "players" lean the puppets and cross on the mirrored walls. Stacey and Judy B. hug a tearful Christy as they take their seats. I find it difficult to speak. I scan the whole group and see other tears. I say this and recognize the power of this dramatic code for all of us, especially for those who enacted it. I ask if any of the presenting group want to share how it felt to do this. Roz said she didn't like being Uncle Sam's right hand. Gentle laughter. Ruth said to Roz that often the right hand had been raised to hurt our people. Roz agreed. Judy said she, too, found it difficult representing Uncle Sam. I explained to the audience that Judy has been jailed for civil disobedience regarding nuclear disarmament, the military budget, and the trident submarine, and asked that she tell us about it. She briefly elaborated as to her reasons for coming to Connecticut as part of the peace movement and the connections between the military budget and homelessness. She also said that the papier mâché puppets were created by Jackie Allen-Doucot, a young woman who works at the MSP Shelter, who also went to jail for civil disobedience. Jackie and her husband, Chris, started a Catholic Worker House in the north end of Hartford near the shelter. I explained that Catholic Worker Houses used some of the same principles as Settlement Houses. The workers lived in the community and shared all they had in reciprocity with community residents, some of whom also lived in the house. Judy B. explained that the cross is a Catholic Worker Cross and that Marley has helped carry it in demonstrations at Electric Boat in Groton where the Trident and Sea Wolf submarines are made. The puppets also go to these demonstrations for street theater. The cost of the nuclear fleet could eradicate homelessness and deflate poverty in the United States.

Gail responded that Judy Beaumont has taught us the activism we speak of in the empowerment approach with her life. She added that taking on the pain of the Mourning Mother is very hard. Stacey said that it is sad to be the Mourning Mother, but it also makes her angry to think that her kids are experiencing a segregated education right here in Hartford. She asked Christy if she was O.K. Christy said that she was but that her life was still heavy at times and she found it hard to talk. I said that today she talked loud and clear by just being here and taking part. She was applauded. Jean shared that because she is white, clients at the Shelter sometimes literally see her as the arm of Uncle Sam. Some think she has caused their troubles and also that she has the power to change things, but the power comes in joining together. Dealing with this in the group is not easy. What helps is when she shares her own struggles to attain empowerment during and after a difficult divorce struggle. She also identifies with the Mourning Mother whose face can be black, yellow, brown, or white, as in Bosnia now. Ruth agreed and added that she has mourned a lot, too, as a mother of six African-American children who are now young adults. Before she was "Dr. Ruth" she was "Mom," and she understands what Christy and Stacey are feeling. I asked Marley and Channel how they were feeling. Marley said "good" and put thumbs up. Channel said tax money should go to make good schools. She added that she liked giving out the big dollars. She enjoyed the applause.

I now turned to the rest of our group, the audience.

The Whole Group at Work

Ella Harris, an African-American woman and administrator of a mental health agency in New York City and also a private practitioner, was the first to address the group. She thanked the group members for presenting this code and tearfully acknowledged that it was difficult for her to share in the experience. Difficult, but so important. In her life and in her many years of practice, she has experienced the pain of prejudice and discrimination. She is moved to tears by the blocked opportunities of her people. The African-American boy on the cross is symbolic of two things to her: all of the young black men who drop out of inadequate schools and wind up in jail or at dead-end jobs or just plain dead; and the faith that enables her and her people to overcome the hatred in this society. There were expressions of solemn agreement all around. Ella noted that she has never seen this degree of honesty and relevance in other conferences. This was a special moment for her. Marcia Cohen of the University of New England in Maine, gave further facts substantiating the structural inequities experienced by poor people in America. Margot Breton said that the code is relevant in Canada and elsewhere as well. Such structural inequity is not limited to the United States. A young woman from Canada elaborated. This was echoed by a participant from Great Britain.

Sunny Abels of The University of California at Long Beach then said that while she appreciated the meaning of the code for the group, she had to add that the symbol of the cross troubled her as it has been an instrument of the oppression of Jews and others throughout history. I welcomed Sunny's concern and said that I was also thinking that if no one said that, I would raise the issue. I was glad she could risk it. I added that anti-semitism was a very real concern these days and right here in Connecticut. Sadly, it may still come from people who call themselves Christians. A student from Connecticut shared incidences of anti-semitism and also anti-Asian, anti-gay, and anti-black activities that occurred at UCONN and elsewhere in the state over the last few years. Another student shared ways in which students at the School of Social Work are fighting such ignorance. A young white man then said that he noticed the names on the cross as it passed: Jesus, Mahatma Gandhi, Ita Ford, Dorothy Day, Martin Luther King Jr. He recognized that they stood for and died for love, action, change, and non-violent civil disobedience. He said that the enactment made him wonder what happened to his own activism. He pays taxes without question. He doesn't fight for the kind of social programs that could make a difference for poor people. He prefers clinical/therapeutic to political skills. In a way, he condones institutional oppression. Perhaps his short-lived interest in activism needs to be reawakened. This is how he decoded the code. Several applauded in agreement.

Another white man said that he wanted to carry the cross for Marley. He realized that he could do that by taking some responsibility for social change, ideally alongside of clients. He noted the heavy load children carry and thanked Marley for helping us see this. Marley beamed. Jean said that it is sometimes particularly difficult to see the sad faces of the children who stay at the shelter. Roz said that seeing them happy at MSPII was a plus. She elaborated on the group work with children at MSPII. Gail said that her group members suffer oppression for their mental illness, in addition to being women and mostly people of color. It is important for oppressed groups not to fight among themselves and to find some common ground. As a staff, we also find community together and that helps us to deal with sometimes difficult practice issues. All agreed.

Judy B. commented on the double and triple jeopardy our clients experience. An African-American woman shared an experience of sexism and racism combined. She complimented the women who presented on their strengths. Roz said that the strengths of the women we work with is what energizes us. She gave a brief example. I asked if either of the members of the Successful Women's Group could comment on their struggles and successes. Stacey said that she has been walking a hard road. While she has made several steps forward, it seems that she also has to take some steps back. She is thankful that her children are growing beautifully and that she has a good job and has advanced in five years. Yet, she is worried about the downsizing and layoffs at her job. Soon, she will have to commute to a different city. What will be next? Will she be laid off and have to start all over again? It is very scary. Ruth said that she knows about the last-to-be-hired and the first-to-be-fired mentality. It is part of African-American history, especially when gains in affirmative action are threatened. I asked Ruth to share her own thoughts and experiences as we drew this experience to a close.

Ending the Presentation: Ruth's Message of Encouragement

Ruth said that she enjoyed being a part of this group of strong women and thanked the group for inviting her. She continued, "This is truly a momentous occasion. When I was first invited as an African 'griot,' I wondered aloud, 'Me, a griot/elder? What can I say that would sound wise and profound? And, weren't the old griots from Africa male, not female?' But then I said to myself, 'Why must men be the norm by which all wise thoughts are measured?'

"As I began to beat the drum, I felt a surge of emotional swelling within my chest. The feeling of marching to the beat of the drum reminded me that this was the language of my forefathers. The tin can that I used for a drum carried a picture of rice growing in a field. This picture carried me back to my early childhood and the memory of my father, for not only did we grow rice on our farm, but my father tried his hand at entrepreneurship (a rice and grits mill, and a saw mill). Even though he was never a complete success, he tried and tried and tried. And always, there were the racial issues as Cornel West affirmed in *Race Matters*, the aim of which was to 'revitalize our public conversation about race,' (p. 158). Years after my father refused to become a sharecropper and declared, 'my children are going to school,' race continued to matter, and education for Negroes was not considered essential. In 1941, after my father had recovered from the Great Depression, he bought a huge farm. He died a year later. Yet, the legacy of the strength to survive continues to this day. Race mattered even after we bought the farm. My perceptions were validated when I read Mays' autobiography (1987), a man born 34 years before me, and found some of the same racial issues. He wrote that 'the Negro who owned land had to be exceedingly careful not to be accused by white people of being uppity.' Further, 'the more a Negro owned, the more humble he had to act in order to keep in the good grace of the white people' (p. 9). This was quite noticeable when we went away to school and returned home on vacation. My mother always insisted that we children come out to speak to Mr. So and So. I felt resentment even though these were white folks who were good to my family. In fact, one gentleman and my father were friends for years. The day of my mother's funeral, the same gentleman parked his tractor and waited with respect as the funeral procession passed. And one other gentleman encouraged me when I was in college. . . .

"Being invited to participate in this empowerment group makes me appreciate my past and helps to strengthen me for the future. Again, I am reminded of the number of times, because of racial struggles, poverty, and inaccessible schooling, I was required to pick myself up, dust off, and start again. I am also reminded of how badly this information is needed in the profession of social work. Racial discrimination continues to be destructive in this country, which means that social workers still need to be trained to recognize and deal with these issues early in the relationship. Stiles and colleagues' "Hear It Like It Is," first published in 1972, is not outdated. It suggests that discussions of race have to become an integral part of social work process with clients/group members. . . .

"All these years as I have worked in the profession of social work, as practitioner and college professor, I have come to understand the full meaning of the need for open and clear communication. I question ways to help my peers understand that the many experiences from my past have made me a solid person, sure of myself, and of my values. My mother always told us, 'You are as good as anybody.' Even though most white people have not acted that way toward me, this I know. And because of that knowledge, as a social worker in the public schools working with a group of white women married to Navy men, I was able to help them deal with their husband's absences while on submarine duties. The women said, 'We believe you like us, Dr. Martin. You never talk down to us, even though we know you are very knowledgeable and must interact with educated people. You always treat us with respect.'

"How do I help a group of white students in the classroom understand that the richness of my life is unique and that there is so much that they can learn? How do I help black students, social workers, and group members understand that you can do this white man's work and our own work? The depth and breadth of what you are is there. Don't give in. Don't give up. Set your sight upon a star and reach. I did it, so can you. I believe this is what it means to be a griot/elder: to help the group to grow and excel."*

CONCLUSION

Dr. Martin then asked the presenting group to rise to a standing ovation. I suggested that we were all clapping for each other in the

---

*A fuller section on Dr. Martin's thoughts and those of other members of the presenting group may be found in "Reflections on Empowerment Group Work Across Racial Lines: My Sisters' Place" by Judith A. B. Lee, Ruth R. Martin, Judith Beaumont, Rosalind Moore-Beckham, Gail Bourdon, Christy King, Jean Konan, and Evelyn Thorpe. In Allan Brown and Tara Mistry (Eds.), *Group Work and Race*. London: Whiting and Birch, Ltd. (Forthcoming.)

effort of mutual empowerment. It was good to reach for that star together. May the work continue!

BIBLIOGRAPHY

Breton, Margot (1992). Liberation theology, group work, and the right of the poor and oppressed to participate in the life of the community. In James A. Garland (Ed.), *Group Work Reaching Out: People, Places and Power.* Binghamton, NY: The Haworth Press. 257-270.

Bricker-Jenkins, Mary and Nancy Hooyman (1986). *Not for women only.* Silver Spring, MD: NASW.

Brown, Allan (1990). British perspectives on group work: present and future. *Social Work with Groups,* 13(3): 35-40.

Chau, Kenneth (1990). Introduction: Facilitating bicultural development and intercultural skills in ethnically heterogeneous groups. In Kenneth Chau (Ed.), *Ethnicity and Biculturalism: Emerging Perspectives of Social Group Work.* Binghamton, NY: The Haworth Press. 1-5.

Coyle, Grace (1930). *Social process in organized groups.* Rpt. Hebron, CT: Practitioners Press, 1979.

Davis, Larry E. (1984). The significance of color. In Larry E. Davis (Ed.), *Ethnicity in Social Group Work Practice.* Binghamton, NY: The Haworth Press. 3-5.

Davis, Larry E. (1984). Essential components of group work with Black Americans. In Larry E. Davis (Ed.), *Ethnicity in Social Group Work Practice.* Binghamton, NY: The Haworth Press. 97-110.

Delgado, Melvin and Denise, Humm-Delgado (1984). Hispanics and group work: A review of the literature. In Larry E. Davis (Ed.), *Ethnicity in Social Group Work Practice.* Binghamton, NY: The Haworth Press. 85-96.

Etter-Lewis, G. (1991). Black women's life stories: reclaiming self in narrative texts. In S.B. Gluck and D. Pataik (Eds.), *Women's Words: The Feminist Practice of Oral History.* New York: Routledge.

Freire, Paulo (1973). *Pedagogy of the oppressed.* New York: Seabury.

Garvin, Charles (1985). Work with disadvantaged and oppressed groups. In Martin Sundel et al. (Eds.), *Individual Change Through Small Groups* (2nd ed.). New York: Free Press. 469-472.

Germain, Carel B. (1991). *Human behavior in the social environment: An ecological view.* New York: Columbia University Press.

Germain, Carel B. and Alex Gitterman (1980). *The life model of social work practice.* New York: Columbia University Press (2nd edition in press).

Gopaul-McNicol, Sharon-Ann (1993). *Working with West Indian Families.* New York: The Guilford Press.

Greene, Beverly (1994). African-American women. In Lillian Comás-Diaz and Beverly Greene (Eds.), *Women of color: Integrating ethnic and gender identities in psychotherapy.* New York: The Guilford Press. 10-29.

Gutiérrez, Lorraine (1991). Empowering women of color: A feminist model. In Mary Bricker-Jenkins, Nancy R. Hooyman, and Naomi Gottlieb (Eds.), *Feminist Social Work Practice in Clinical Settings*. Plenary Speech, 17th AASWG Symposium, San Diego California, October 27, 1995. Newbury Park, CA: Sage. 199-214.

Gutiérrez, Lorraine and Robert Ortega (1989). Using groups to empower Latinos: A preliminary analysis. In *Proceedings of the Eleventh Annual Symposium*. Akron, OH: AASWG.

hooks, bell (1990). *Yearning: Race, gender, and cultural politics*. Boston: South End Press.

Hull, G., P.B., Scott, and B. Smith (1982) (Eds.), *All the women are white, and all the blacks are men, but some of us are brave: Black women's studies*. Old Westbury, NY: The Feminist Press.

Konopka, Gisela (1988). *Courage and love*. Edina, MN: Burgess

Lang, Norma (1986). Social work practice in small social forms: Identifying collectively. In Norma Lang and Joanne Sullivan (Eds.), *Collectively in Social Group Work*. Binghamton, NY: The Haworth Press.

Lee, Judith A.B. (ed.) (1989). *Group work with the poor and oppressed*. New York: Haworth.

Lee, Judith A.B. (1991). Empowerment through mutual aid groups: A practice grounded conceptual framework. *Group Work* 4(1): 5-21.

Lee, Judith A.B. (1992). Jane Addams in Boston: Intersecting time and space. In James A. Garland (Ed.), *Group Work Reaching Out: People, Places and Power*. Binghamton, NY: The Haworth Press. 7-22.

Lee, Judith A.B. (1994a). *The empowerment approach to social work practice*. New York: Columbia University Press.

Lee, Judith A.B. (1994b). No place to go: Homeless women. In Alex Gitterman and Lawrence Shulman (Eds.), *Mutual Aid Groups, Vulnerable Populations, and the Life Cycle*. New York: Columbia University Press. 297-313.

Lum, Doman (1995). *Social work practice and people of color* (3rd edition.). Monterey, CA: Brook-Cole.

Martin, Ruth (1994). *Oral history in social work: Research, assessment, and intervention*. Thousand Oaks, CA: Sage.

Mays, B.E. (1987). *Born to rebel: An autobiography*. Athens, GA: The University of Georgia Press.

Mistry, Tara (1995). 1994 Hartford Symposium. *Group Work* 8(1): 99-101.

Mullender, Audrey (1990). The ebony project–Bicultural group work with transracial foster parents. *Social Work with Groups* 13(4): 23-42.

Mullender, Audrey and David Ward. *Self-directed group work: Users take action for empowerment*. London, England: Whiting and Birch, Ltd.

Papell, Catherine P. and Beulah Rothman (1980). Relating the mainstream model of social work with groups. *Social Work with Groups*, 3(summer): 5-22.

Parsons, Ruth (1991). Empowerment: Purpose and practice principles in social work. *Social Work with Groups* 14(2): 7-21.

Pence, Ellen (1987). *In our best interests: A process for personal and social change*. Deluth, MN: Minnesota Program Development.

Pernell, Ruby (1986). Empowerment and social group work. In Marvin Parnes (Ed.), *Innovations in Social Group Work*. Binghamton, NY: The Haworth Press. 107-118.

Schwartz, William (1974). The social worker in the group. In Robert W. Klenk and Robert W. Ryan (Eds.), *The Practice of Social Work* (2nd ed.). Belmont, CA: Wadsworth. 208-228.

Solomon, Barbara B. (1976). *Black empowerment: Social work in oppressed communities*. New York: Columbia University Press.

Stiles, E., S. Donner, J. Giovannone, E. Lochte, and R.R. Reetz (1982). Hear it like it is. In H. Rubenstein, and M.H. Bloch (Eds.), *Things That Matter*. New York: Macmillan Publishing Co., Inc.

West, Cornel (1993). *Race matters*. Boston, MA: Beacon Press.

Wood, Gale Goldberg and Ruth Middleman (1989). *The structural approach to social work practice*. New York: Columbia University Press.

Wood, Gale Goldberg and Ruth Middleman (1995). Constructivism, power and social work with groups. *Plenary Speech*, 17th AASWG Symposium, San Diego, California, October 27, 1995.

Chapter 4

When Worker and Member Expectations Collide: The Dilemma of Establishing Group Norms in Conflictual Situations

Roselle Kurland
Robert Salmon

INTRODUCTION

The development of positive norms is crucial to a group's success. Norms that encourage respect, openness, honesty, support, mutual aid, acceptance of difference, experimentation, and flexibility contribute mightily to group cohesion and to group and individual growth and development. (See, for example, Glassman and Kates, 1990.) Yet the establishment of positive norms is increasingly difficult today when the environment in which many groups exist is filled with behavioral expectations that are in opposition to the norms that have been valued traditionally in group work.

Though the group work literature acknowledges that there can be conflict between the values of a particular group and those of other groups or of the larger community, as well as wide disparity between the expectations that a worker has for the group's members and those of the members themselves (Northen, 1988; Balgopal and Vassil, 1983), little is said about group work practice when such situations occur. Increasingly, group workers are confronted by such conflict around norms, reflecting the erosion of traditional societal values, roles, and relationships and the increasing violence

43

and despair of group life that have occurred during the past four decades (Vigilante, 1983; Kurland and Salmon, 1992b). The disparity of norms between worker and member and/or worker and agency has widened and created difficult practice dilemmas.

This chapter will examine those practice dilemmas, which are faced by workers in establishing group norms when there is a disparity between the norms that the worker hopes to develop and those that seem to be valued by the group members, their friends, families, and cultural reference groups, and/or by the agencies in which the group takes place. Implications for group work practice will be identified and discussed.

EXPOSITION

All groups develop norms—what it is OK to do and not OK to do in the group, (Middleman and Wood, 1990), ways in which group members expect each other to behave and to be. Northen's definition (1988) is comprehensive.

> A norm is a generalization concerning an expected standard of behavior in any matter of consequence to the group. It incorporates a value judgment. It is a standard to which the members of the group expect each other to adhere . . . A set of norms defines the range of behavior that will be tolerated within the group and introduces a certain amount of predictability in the group's functioning because members feel some obligation to adhere to the expectations of the group, which they have had a part in developing. A norm implies that certain rewards and sanctions will be invoked for conformity to or deviation from the norms of the group. (p. 33)

Balgopal and Vassil (1983) describe norms as ideas that guide behavior and that are maintained through sanctions such as ridicule from others and self-guilt. Similarly, Homans describes group norms as "ideas in the minds of members about what should and should not be done by a specific member under specified circumstances" (1950, p. 123). Middleman and Wood (1990) note that norms provide boundaries and limits to a group's activities and enable the group to conduct its "business" in an orderly manner.

The worker plays a major role in helping the group to develop norms. (See, for example, Northen, 1988; Shulman, 1992; Brown, 1991; Balgopal and Vassil, 1983; Glassman and Kates, 1990). His or her own actions in the group are a model for group members of behavior that the worker deems appropriate and inappropriate. In addition to modelling appropriate behavior, the worker supports some behaviors of group members and withholds support for other behaviors, thereby having an important influence in the process of norm development. At other times, the worker helps the group establish norms by setting limits on member behavior and/or by pointing out to the group the ways in which they seem to prefer to do things. At still other times, the worker may influence the group's establishment of norms by teaching the members to do something in a certain way (Northen, 1988).

Through modelling, supporting, limiting, and teaching, it is the worker who has a major influence in determining what the group's norms will be. His or her beliefs, based on the values of the profession (see NASW Code of Ethics, 1980) and on his or her own personal values as well, are quite central in creating group norms. That is not to say that group members do not have input into creating group norms or that the worker can impose upon a group ways of behaving that are unacceptable to the group members. But group members are usually open to the influence of the worker, and those norms that have been traditionally at the heart of group work practice are often welcomed by the group members, even when they may entail ways of behaving that are new to them.

Increasingly, however, workers are encountering situations in which the norms of behavior that members bring into the group differ from those that the worker wants to establish. It is difficult, for example, to establish norms of mutual respect and acceptance of difference in groups with teenagers whose lives on the streets are filled with hair-trigger violence and communication through "dissing" and put-downs.

Consider, for example, the following conversation among the members of a new group of eighth graders in a public school, discussing difficulties they have in getting along with their parents:

Maria was talking quite animatedly about how strict her parents were, complaining that her mother does not allow her to stay out past 10:00 p.m. even on weekends. "You probably need that, whore," Jake shouted from across the room. The group laughed. "Shut up, puerca (pig)," Maria shot back to Jake. "Fuck you," he said in return. "That's exactly what *you* need, a good fuck–but you're a homo," Lisa, who was Maria's friend, said to Jake. Jake made an obscene gesture in return. Joann, the worker, asked Maria to continue. "I have nothing more to say," Maria said, turning around in her chair so that her back was to the group.

"Dissing," put-downs, sharp and quick insults back and forth characterized the way in which teens related to one another throughout the school in which this group took place. The group members brought that way of relating into this group. Establishing norms of respect, honesty, and support among the group members will be difficult when relationships that are characterized by those qualities are so very far from the ways in which these teens are used to relating to each other–when they seem to value and afford prestige and status to the cleverest insulter and the person who can shoot off the slickest retorts. Norms that the group members seem to value and that are prevalent in their peer group and in their lives outside the group clash with those the worker wishes to see established as characteristic of members' behavior in the group.

At other times, norms of members' cultural reference groups may seem to clash with the group norms that the worker wishes to establish. Honesty and openness in discussion may be difficult to achieve when, for example, members' cultures hold that personal problems should not be aired in public or when the belief is that difficulties and problems should stay within and be able to be addressed within the family. Similarly, when cultural values maintain that discussion of sex in public is a taboo, establishing norms of honesty and openness around such discussion may not be possible. Culturally and family-based beliefs, values, and taboos will be brought into the group by its members and may challenge the establishment of norms valued by the worker. For example,

Susan had been working with a group of sixth graders in a community center after-school program. The group met twice a week. All the girls were Latina. Susan was of Italian background. Because she walked the girls home after the group meetings, Susan had gotten to know the girls' parents as she often talked with them informally when she dropped their daughters off. After meeting with the group for three months, it became apparent to Susan that the group members knew little about sex, had many myths and misconceptions, and were curious about it. She thought it would be a good idea to use some of the group meetings for sex education and wanted the girls' parents to know she planned to do this in the group. As she talked with the parents about this, most thought it was a good idea. But the parents of three of the girls were adamant that she not do so. "Absolutely not," Mrs. Ramos said. "You don't talk about sex in public." Similarly, Mrs. Garcia said, "I don't want my daughter doing that. I won't let her stay in the group if that's what you're going to do." And Mrs. Alonso also did not want her daughter to talk about sex in the group. "She can talk to me if she wants," she told Susan, "but I don't want her talking about sex with strangers."

Agency norms are also crucial. They, too, have an important impact upon a group, and they, too, may differ from norms that the worker hopes to see a group establish. Acceptance of and respect for difference, for example, are difficult norms to achieve in a group that is part of an agency in which the expression of conflict seems to be discouraged and frowned upon. The agency's norms, like those of the peer and cultural reference groups, will affect members' group participation. For example,

A group of visually impaired, emotionally disturbed young adults in a day treatment program were talking about their goals. Alvin was saying that sighted people have some of the same problems that visually impaired people do. Suddenly, Sonia stood up and said she was going to leave the group. Martha, the worker, who had been at the agency for only two months, urged Sonia to take her seat, telling her that what was bothering her could be talked about in the group. "No, it

can't," Sonia said. "It's personal. I'm mad. I'm mad at someone in this group." Martha responded, "Well then, we can talk
about what you are angry about in the group. It's OK to talk
about things even when we are upset." Carla, another group
member, responded, "I don't know if you know it Martha, but
we have a rule about not fighting or arguing in group." Do-
lores, another member, added, "That's right, Martha. We're
not supposed to argue in group. If two people argue, it's only
between those two people and not the business of everybody."
Irv agreed, "Roger (the program's director) says we're supposed to go to our social worker, that there are to be no fighting or arguments in group."

In this group, the members' understanding of the program's attitude
toward conflict and the expression of interpersonal difference is in
direct opposition to the norms regarding the expression, appreciation,
and acceptance of difference that the worker wants to encourage.

What, then, does the worker do when there is a conflict between the
norms that he or she hopes the group will establish and those of the
group members? The steps the worker needs to take closely parallel
the steps in the problem-solving process formulated by John Dewey
(1910). Following recognition of the difficulty, Dewey advised identifying and exploring the problem or issue, considering alternative solutions, deciding on a solution to try, implementing the decision, and
then evaluating the results. This process is applicable when the issue or
problem is a difference between worker and members around norms.

Five practice principles pertain to and need to be applied in situations where norms seem to differ. First, the worker needs to identify
the areas of seeming difference between him or herself and the group
members in the norms that are preferred. The worker also needs to
identify the source(s) of the members' preferences. Are the norms
coming from the behaviors, values, beliefs, and/or points of view of
the members' peer group, their families and/or cultural reference
groups, or the agency in which the group takes place? Such consideration will enable the worker to determine with whom it is best to
discuss the situation—the members themselves, others who influence
the members, or agency administrators.

For example, further discussing whether conflict is to be expressed or discussed in the day treatment group of visually impaired young adults cited earlier, when the "message" in the larger program is that conflicts are *not* to be addressed in groups, would be unfair to the group members. It would place them in the center of a difference that more accurately needs to be worked out between the worker and the program's director.

Similarly, asking the sixth graders at the community center to speak openly and honestly about sex when their norm is to not do so in their families and when some of their parents actively disapprove of their doing so would also place them in the center of a difference that needs to be first worked out between the worker and the parents of the girls.

On the other hand, asking the members of the eighth grade group in the school how they wish to treat and relate to one another would be quite appropriate. That decision is one that the group members themselves need to make, and in that group the difference in norms is between the worker and the group members directly.

Second, the worker needs to take the time to understand the point of view of those who espouse norms that seem to be different from those that he or she might prefer. To gain such understanding, the worker needs to skillfully explore with the group members or with their families and significant others or with agency administrators the values and beliefs that shape those norms. The thoughts and feelings of those with views that are different from the worker's own need to have a chance to be expressed. The worker needs to encourage such expression. Furthermore, the worker needs to be open to the possibility that greater understanding of the views of others may bring about greater acceptance of their viewpoints on his or her part and a change in his or her own thinking and preferences. (For a discussion of this, see Kurland and Salmon, 1992a.)

Third, the worker needs to challenge the views of the members, families, or agency administrators if, after they have had a chance to express their points of view in regard to the norms under question, the worker continues to believe that those norms would not be best for the group. The worker's aim here is not to impose his or her own viewpoint, but rather to really encourage the members, families, or administrators to stop and think about the views they are expressing. Knowing that the worker understands and has taken the time to learn about their views leaves group members, parents, or administrators much more open to the worker's challenge of them (Kurland and Salmon, 1992a).

In all three of the examples cited here, discussion of norms and challenges from the worker were important steps. Frank discussion with the eighth graders of the "dissing" phenomenon unearthed the fact that they actually disliked and were frequently hurt by it, but felt they would lose face in the eyes of their peers if they did not engage in "dissing."

When Susan, the social worker with the sixth graders, discovered that some parents did not want sex to be discussed in the group, she called a parents meeting to discuss the issue. Parents who were in favor of their daughters' discussing sex in the group were effective in convincing the parents who were initially opposed that such discussion was a good idea. Although Susan's desire to open the topic in the group did not change, she emerged from the parents meeting with a clear sense of the parents' concerns and ideas about ways to raise the subject with the girls.

Martha, the worker in the day treatment program, discussed the subject of conflict with the program's director. She discovered that the group members had misunderstood what the program director had said to them about conflict—that it was, in fact, not a taboo of the program. She also discovered that conflictual situations in groups in the past had resulted in great upset for the clients, and even in violence in one instance. This population of clients, she learned, does have difficulty managing disagreements, and conflict needs to be approached with care with them, moreso than she had realized.

Fourth, the group members, with the help of the worker, need to make a decision about how they will handle the norm under question. If discussion with others, such as parents or agency administrators, has taken place, then this needs to be reported to the group members.

For example, once the phenomenon of "dissing" was discussed in the eighth-grade group and the worker expressed directly to the group her preference for norms of respect, honesty, and support along with the reasons for her preference, the group members said they would try not to put each other down all the time. This was going to be new for them, they warned the worker, and might be difficult. But, they said, they liked the idea of not having to constantly keep their "guard" up and were willing to give it a try.

In the sixth-grade group, the members seemed relieved to learn that discussion of sex would take place with the knowledge and approval of their parents. Some of the members said they had been worried that they would have to hide the fact of the group's discussions from their parents, and they did not want to do that. The sense of the worker was that norms of honesty and openness would now be more possible in the group.

Similarly in the day-treatment group, the members seemed relieved to learn that the worker had discussed with the program director whether differences and disagreements could be expressed in the group. With this population, for whom limits and structure are important, agreement between the worker and the program director provided needed reassurance. The group members were now free to work toward norms of acceptance of and respect for difference.

Finally, when the norms *in* the group differ for the members from those *outside* the group, the worker needs to acknowledge his or her awareness of that. Such differences in in-group and out-group norms need to be made explicit and discussed in the group. Such discussion may strengthen members' adherence to the group's norms and result in greater group cohesiveness. Schwartz' view (1971, 1976) of the social worker as mediator is especially relevant here. If the worker indicates his or her understanding to be that norms for the members in and out of the group are different, then group members know that they can discuss in the group those differences and the conflicts that result for them in their lives outside the group. Such discussions may help group members negotiate other conflicts between themselves and "the various systems through which they carry on their relationship with society" (Schwartz, 1976, p. 184).

Ultimately, discussion of such conflicts in norms may help affect the behavior of group members when they are away from the group (Hartford, 1971). The group of eighth graders provides a particularly good example of a group where discussions of conflict between group and outside norms would be especially important and valuable.

CLOSING STATEMENT

"The highest form of human society is that in which the desire to do what is best for the whole dominates and limits the action of every member of that society" (T. H. Huxley, 1893, p. 53). In the kind of society proposed by T. H. Huxley in 1903, norms of behavior would be understood, uniform, and effective due to agreement on the goal of working toward the common good. However, that happy and ideal situation does not exist and, in fact, group workers increasingly face sharply disparate norms among the groups they lead and the systems in which they find themselves. For instance, it has been noted that there is increasing conflict between the policies of social agencies and the professional values of workers (Vigilante, 1983). As a result, conflict of norms may be cause for great stress in these situations as workers are called upon to mediate the impossible (Lewis, 1980). Intense frustration and burnout often develop.

However, there is much that is positive that can be accomplished as the worker plans and undertakes work with the group. Change may be incremental, but it is important. Addressing the disparity of norms in order to help the group achieve its purpose is the desired outcome that can result from skillful intervention here. It also is important as it will provide workers with a major focus for their work in a difficult social environment. This paper has provided an approach for their efforts and some of the tools workers can use as they undertake the task.

REFERENCES

Balgopal, Pallasana and Vassil, Thomas. (1983) *Groups in Social Work: An Ecological Perspective*, Macmillan Publishing Co., Inc.

Brown, Leonard N. (1991) *Groups for Growth and Change*, Longman.

Dewey, John. (1910) *How We Think*, Heath.

Glassman, Urania and Kates, Len. (1990) *Group Work: A Humanistic Approach*, Sage Publications.

Hartford, Margaret. (1971) *Groups in Social Work*, Columbia University Press.

Homans, George. (1950) *The Human Group*, Harcourt Brace.

Huxley, Thomas H. (1893) *Science and Christian Tradition*, D. Appleton and Company.

Kurland, Roselle and Salmon, Robert. (1992a) "Self-Determination: Its Use and Misuse in Group Work Practice and Social Work Education," in David Fike and Barbara Rittner (Eds.), *Working from Strengths: The Essence of Group Work*, Center for Group Work Studies.

Kurland, Roselle and Salmon, Robert. (1992b) "When Problems Seem Overwhelming: Emphases in Teaching, Supervision, and Consultation," *Social Work*, 37(3).

Lewis, Harold. (1980) "The Battered Helper," *Child Welfare*, 59(4).

Middleman, Ruth and Wood, Gale Goldberg. (1990) *Skills for Direct Practice in Social Work*, Columbia University Press.

NASW Code of Ethics. (1980) *Social Work*, 25(3).

Northen, Helen. (1988) *Social Work with Groups*, Columbia University Press.

Schwartz, William. (1971) "On the Use of Groups in Social Work Practice," in William Schwartz and Serapio Zalba (Eds.), *The Practice of Group Work*, Columbia University Press.

Schwartz, William. (1976) "Between Client and System: The Mediating Function," in Robert W. Roberts and Helen Northen, (Eds.), *Theories of Social Work With Groups*, Columbia University Press.

Shulman, Lawrence. (1992) *The Skills of Helping Individuals, Families and Groups*, F.E. Peacock Publishers.

Vigilante, Joseph. (1983) "Professional Values," in Aaron Rosenblatt and Diana Waldfogel (Eds.), *Handbook of Clinical Social Work*, Jossey-Bass Publishers.

Chapter 5

Group Work
with Juvenile Sex Offenders

Kym Crown
Dan Gates

As improved reporting of sexual offenses against children brings
more and more sexual offenders into the justice system, there is a
greater need for effective treatment options for this population.
There has been much research on the efficacy of psychotherapy for
reducing sexually offending behavior, especially in adults. Outcome studies affirming one treatment method over another are difficult to design. However, recent studies suggest that cognitive behavioral approaches in group settings work better than individual,
insight-oriented methods (Marshall, Laws, and Barbaree, 1989).
This chapter proposes a model for working with male sex offenders
between the ages of 14 and 20 who can be treated on an outpatient
basis. These young people are not exhibiting addictions to drugs,
psychotic thought process, or antisocial behavior that requires insti-
tutionalization for the safety of the community. They also have at
least borderline intellectual functioning. This chapter examines the
program design, goals of treatment, and the reasons as well as the
problems with the techniques and modalities of treatment.

THEORETICAL ORIENTATION

The assumption made concerning why juvenile sex offenders
commit such acts is that although there is secondary gain in sexual

pleasure, the primary purpose is to control another. The feeling behind this need varies. It may be the result of rage and/or power-lessness. It may be a need to humiliate others so as to not experience his own feelings of humiliation at the hands of those older and more powerful than himself. Research indicates that offenders are no more likely to have been victims of sex offenders than anyone else in the population. It is also assumed that sexual offenses are self-reinforcing because they meet several needs at once. The offender can experience sexual pleasure, experience control over another, and can experience a number of other wants being gratified. There is often a profound sense of emptiness in these youths, which is filled while they are sexually offending. It gives them a sense of excitement and control in the secrecy that they must maintain and that they induce their victims to maintain. Although it is believed that sexual abuse does not create an offender, these youths all have dysfunctional relationships with their families and have great pain. They find a solution to that pain in sexual offenses against children significantly younger than themselves.

These adolescents are unable to report their internal feelings usually, and are completely unconscious of their own motivation. In fact, they frequently report they did not think what they were doing was hurting their victim. They usually have a number of ways to rationalize and minimize their behavior, such as, "I only did it once," or, "I would have stopped it if she told me to."

Providing treatment to this population is extremely challenging. Initially, there is no internal reason to stop the behavior. Sexual offenses meet their needs. There are only external reasons to stop, like being arrested, like embarrassing and hurting their families, like being removed from their homes. So following this logic, one answer would be for them to hide it more effectively. This solution is not lost on the minds of perpetrators. The second challenge is that they don't often feel they need therapy to stop offending. They can simply stop. They do not have insight into the fact that when they are caught, the feeling state that they were in when they were offending is no longer present. But it will return when they are no longer in the crisis of being discovered. The third challenge is that they are juveniles, so they have the same grandiosity that many adolescents have, thinking that if adults would simply leave them alone, they would be able to manage themselves. They rarely start the program without resentment about having to come to therapy. So first, some kind of alliance must be created with them. They must like the practitioner and must feel liked by him or her so there is a reason to cooperate. Second, guilt must be induced to motivate a behavior change so there is an internalized reason to stop offending, as the external reasons may not be enough after the initial crisis passes. After that, a combination of cognitive and behavioral methods as well as an affective component is necessary for the perpetrator to be able to acknowledge his feelings, deal with them in a more appropriate way, and develop a plan for what to do if and when he has the urge to re-offend. He also needs to make some kind of restitution to his victim, if possible, so that he can begin to develop self-esteem and gain a sense of completion. This program attempts to meet both cognitive and affective challenges. In short, the program must create a safe place for the offender to be so that he can allow the program to break down his coping skills to manage self-esteem issues and make him feel bad about himself by inducing guilt. Then the program must give him a way to develop other methods of gaining self esteem that are more socially acceptable, such as making up for what he did and taking responsibility for himself.

PROGRAM DESIGN

This program meets once a week for an hour and a half. Three weeks out of the month, the modality is group work with the offenders with one clinician. The fourth week of the month is a multi-family meeting that includes the offenders and at least one of their parents, although both parents and any stepparents or other adults living in the home are invited to attend. It is facilitated by a male and female co-therapy team. The group is limited to a maximum of five offenders. It is an ongoing group so membership changes periodically. However, many of the young men are court ordered to stay in the program for between one and two years. Members may be court ordered or may come voluntarily. Usually if they are voluntary, they are being pressured by the victim or the victim's family or their own family if a disclosure has been made. No referrals have been received from a sex offender asking for help who has not been caught. So there is some level of coercion for each of them to enter the program.

Offenders, as well as their parent or guardian, are required to sign a contract in order to be accepted into the program. The contract states that the offender will abide by the rules of the program, which are that attendance is mandatory, payment must be up-to-date unless other arrangements are made, and offenders will participate in the program. Parents agree to come to family meetings and to help their child refrain from further sexually deviant behavior. The purpose of the contract is twofold. The first is to make sure there is no miscommunication about what is expected of both the adolescents and their guardians. The second is to set the tone of the program. The implication is that the staff takes sex offenses very seriously. There is also the connotation that the clinicians do not believe the youths will stop offending solely because they have been caught. The last point is that the clinicians are in charge of the program, and not the participants.

Sessions with only the boys are a combination of education and structured group therapy. The cognitive goals for this phase of treatment are met by the following: the offenders need to know the laws regarding sexually-offensive behavior for the state in which they live; they must be able to identify ways in which they can minimize their behaviors and be able to recognize minimization by others; and they must be able to identify the difference between sexual experimentation and sexually deviant behavior. They are taught the laws regarding sexual offenses, and they are taught what minimization is using the typology of "thinking errors" developed by Samenow and Yochelson. They are also taught what victims who have been sexually abused feel. Stories from victims, visits to the group by victims, and explanations of why victims respond to abuse passively are used. Development of victim empathy is instrumental in inducing guilt. The affective part is met by learning to identify feelings within themselves. The clinician often will help the individual name the feelings, as in any good therapy. Attempts are also made to identify what feelings were being acted out during the sexual offenses and how they might find more appropriate channels and expression for those feelings. The goal is for them to understand what it was in themselves that brought them to commit sexual offenses.

The last part of the program is a monthly family meeting that includes each adolescent and at least one parent or guardian. There are a number of goals that are met by this meeting. It is very traumatizing for families to have their children accused of such an egregious crime. The group offers mutual support and advice from parent to parent about the emotional and legal situations in which these families find themselves. It gives parents a place to process their own hatred, guilt, confusion, and sadness. These families are often deeply entrenched in their own dysfunction, and the crisis created by the discovery that an adolescent in the family is a sex offender often reduces the level of functioning in already marginal families. However, because there are often other problems between these adolescents and their caretakers, they are able to listen to others talk about problems and gain a different perspective. It is also a place where adolescents can see how group leaders deal with their parents. And, it helps the clinicians better understand the environment in which the youths live. Often, events in the multi-family group are processed in the offender group for several weeks after the meeting. Attempts are made to understand the dynamics between parents and children, although no attempts are undertaken to change these dynamics. Such endeavors have failed in the past. It is believed that the families are not sufficiently committed to be willing to change the underlying dynamics. Also, adolescents still need their parents so no emancipation from them, emotional or physical, is recommended unless the situation is dire.

TECHNIQUES WITH THE OFFENDER GROUP

Group leaders must be responsible for establishing group norms and must guide interaction much more than is common in support groups or personal growth groups. The purpose of the groups is not empowerment or for these perpetrators to feel better about themselves. The first goal is for them to come to terms with the reality that they hurt someone else in order to meet their own needs. They usually have tremendous denial toward what they did as being bad. So, therapy makes them feel worse, as they must come to the realization that they are hurtful, selfish, and, in some cases, are criminals. They don't like to think of themselves in these ways.

Like everyone, they prefer to think of themselves as basically good and will concoct elaborate explanations and rationalizations to explain their sexual behavior. Because the work is painful for them and diminishes their ego, they must experience tremendous support from the group in order to tolerate the pain of looking at themselves, especially as none of them chose therapy for themselves. So, despite the authoritarian stance of the clinician, the group must be a place where a sense of belonging and a sense of acceptance of the person is fostered. The goal is for each individual to feel as if his denial is not accepted, but he is accepted and respected as a person. Group norms must be established around this principle.

Techniques used are designed to both increase a sense of belonging in the group and to increase guilt through victim empathy, knowledge of the law, and confrontation of minimization. Support and confrontation must come from the adolescents themselves as well as the group leader. Group members are asked how they are doing and if there are any issues they want to bring up at the beginning of group. They rarely volunteer anything at this time, especially in the beginning stages of treatment, so they are encouraged. Because of the nature of the group, it is assumed that the clinician must take responsibility for "pulling teeth." The clinician asks general questions, such as how is school, relationships with parents, or how did they feel about the last family meeting. Although the attitude is patient, they are each asked specific questions to enhance discussion. When they are able to talk about what is on their minds, the focus moves to identifying feelings about the issues. It is through the discussion of feelings that the issues that brought them to sexually offend are woven into the conversation. Hypothetical situations are mentioned, such as, "It sounds like you are really angry at your Dad because he pushed you around. I am wondering if there was any feeling of anger like that anger when you abused your cousin." The conversation often extends into discussions of feelings about parents, relationships with females, or other issues. It is in these conversations that two things happen. One is that the closeness necessary for the therapeutic work is created. The other is that links between nonoffending-feeling states are related to offending-feeling states; it is an introduction to the concept of their offenses having to do with a feeling about something else in their lives.

Teaching youth to confront one another in a respectful way is an ongoing process. One method used is the technique of practicing cognitive learning on each other. For example, the group leader may ask one member to relate what happened when he sexually offended. He will then ask others in the group to comment on thinking errors they heard, once they have been taught what thinking errors are. They are encouraged and supported for being able to recognize them in others. At the same time, the youth who was relating his story is treated with utmost respect and is thanked for his contribution. There is a great desire on the part of group members to collude with each other's minimization. For example, "I agree with Sam that she was a bitch for gming along with it and then telling on him," or, "He asked her if he could touch her breasts, why was it wrong?" There are a number of reasons why it feels better to collude with minimization. For one thing, it reduces the colluder's culpability. For another, it creates an alliance with a group member based on defining sexual abuse as behaving acceptably, rather than unacceptably. And third, it sets up a power struggle over group norms with the clinician, who is controlling the group norms. Luckily, there are a few factors upon which the clinician can call to reduce the likelihood of this happening. First, there is often at least one member who is starting to feel proud of himself because he has the courage to face what he has done wrong and rectify it. His opinion of the situation can be requested. Also, because the clinician has been central all along, he can exert authority that has already been established. "We are not even going to address whether she is a bitch. It is not the point. What about you?" or, "Who here can tell me why it is wrong? If you can't remember, I will help you." It is important to have more than two group members at any given time, as it is much easier for them to form a stable alliance against the clinician than when there are more members and the relationships between them are constantly changing.

The type of work done in this group often raises the level of anxiety for everyone in the room, so the problem of focus is a constant. Often the youths do not want to pay attention or the conversation will break down. Methods of dealing with this are to have specific projects that are cognitive in nature and can be called upon whenever the anxiety level gets to be too much for the offenders to tolerate. Disciplinary action is avoided, as that sets a punitive tone that simply makes the offenders withdraw emotionally and reduces the supportive atmosphere. Attempts are constantly made to reduce the resentment about being in the program, so unpleasant interchanges in the room are avoided.

The clinicians have all of the problems and advantages of working with adolescents. Adolescents have a high degree of interest in each other. They have a lot of energy. They are more interested in their own norms than they are in the norms of adults. The clinician also has all the problems related to a coerced population and must respect the fact that they do not think that they need to come and do not want to come for treatment as a sex offender. That is not to say that they do not want to get something out of the program. It only means that without an understanding that they do not *want* to recover, the clinicians will become ineffective and will probably burn out. The clinician must also deal with the unique problems of sexual offenders. The techniques offered here are designed to meet all three of the variables that make this population unique.

TECHNIQUES WITH THE MULTIFAMILY GROUP

The multifamily group is a different group from the adolescent group. It has different membership, different goals, and a different lifecycle. Although the two groups are connected, it is important to keep their differences in mind. Because it only meets monthly, it takes members a lot longer to become comfortable with one another. It also is coercive, so there is tremendous resistance on the part of parents to be open, and they often are angry about having to come when they are not the ones who committed the crime. In the beginning, they do not really understand what the purpose of the multi-family group is, so it is important for the facilitators to have a central role in guiding the direction in which the group goes. Unlike the adolescent group, education is not used to reduce anxiety and affect cognitive understanding. Parents are often asked how they are dealing with their sons and later, in treatment, are often asked what they need from the meeting for that particular night. There is a delicate balance that must be maintained between removing any responsibility for the meeting from the participants and allowing them to simply avoid any difficult issues, a common desire in this population. One method used is to ask a parent or adolescent to comment on another parent/child interaction. For example, a parent may say that he is unsure whether or not his son is getting anything out of the program because he refuses to talk about what goes on in the adolescent group. The parent may be encouraged to ask his son right there. The son may answer evasively, or simply say "yes." Another adolescent may be asked to comment on the interaction, and might say that it doesn't look like the son wants to tell the parent too much. The facilitator might ask the second adolescent to hypothesize on why that might be the case. If the youth can't think of any reason, he might be encouraged to confer with the other adolescents to see if any of them have any ideas about this. Usually someone has some ideas, and often other parents will spontaneously respond with their own ideas, especially if they think the adolescents cannot come up with any ideas. This type of intervention will often spark a spontaneous discussion between parents who have the same experience with their children. Eventually, the facilitators will bring the discussion back around to the original parent's question of how to find out how his child is doing in the adolescent group. There is always an attempt to have a positive outcome to questions of this nature in order to encourage parents to bring in more questions and to develop a sense of trust in the group process so they will want to participate in a deeper and more genuine way. It also encourages other parents who are watching what the facilitator does with these kinds of questions. When they see that attempts are made to get answers and to treat such questions with respect, it also encourages them. Attempts are made to give each family some time and attention during the meeting, so the families are aware that they will be given individual attention and will be asked to bring up a problem or concern. Because that becomes a group norm, they plan for it. Sometimes parents will want to avoid difficulties by talking about how well their child has been doing, or asking the facilitators if they want to see the adolescent in his school play, for example. When this happens, parents are often asked if they feel as if their child doesn't have a problem with sexual deviancy if he does well in school or in other arenas of life.

Neither parents nor their adolescents are expected to confront one another in the multi-family group. There is not enough trust that can develop here to expect it. Parents and their kids must ride home with one another after the group so whatever happens in group is something they must deal with at home. Support is expected and often must be guided. Parents who have been in the program for some time are encouraged and even asked to address the concerns of newly arrived parents. But confrontation is up to the facilitators, usually. Sometimes, when families have been in the program for some period of time, they may spontaneously point out flaws in the thinking of another member. Or one parent may tell another's child that he is not looking at the whole picture or is not thinking about the future. They take their cues about how to do this from the facilitators, so it is important for the facilitators to be consistently respectful and positive.

A technique commonly used is for one facilitator to comment to the other about what he or she sees, rather than speaking directly to the person involved. For example, one father consistently bullied his son. He believed that his son had only "experimented with sex" when he had molested a three-year-old cousin. A facilitator asked the adolescent to explain to his father why it was not sexual exper- imentation. When it was clear that this approach was not fruitful, the other facilitator broke into the conversation and told the first facilitator that the youth could not do as he was asked because the youth knew that the father would not listen to him. The two facilita- tors argued back and forth with one another about whether the youth should try to make his father understand. Finally, the father interrupted and insisted that he was quite capable of listening and that his son should go ahead. It is believed that if the conversation about whether the father would listen had been between the boy and his father, it would have been ineffective. Because it was between the two facilitators, the confrontation of the father was indirect. Nothing was being asked of the father, thus, respecting that the father had no personal investment in even being in the group. The father was free to participate in his own time.

Working with the multifamily group requires that the clinicians create an environment that makes participants want to participate in a meaningful way. They must be supportive and respectful of the coercive element operating in the group. But, they must also confront minimization and denial. They must be able to address subjects of family dysfunction, so the offenders can start to develop insight into what happens between them and their parents. There is a great push among therapists to want to work toward changing the dysfunctional patterns they see before them in these families. It is a constant challenge to avoid doing that, unless the family specifically asks for that type of help. In six years, we have met a few families who told us they wanted help changing their dysfunctional patterns. We have had two families who wanted to do it once they learned what was required of them in order to change. So, they occasionally develop a desire to really be in therapy, but it is rare, in our experience.

CONCLUSION

There have been no re-arrests for sexual crimes in the forty perpetrators we have treated over six years. Some of the youths seemed to have turned their lives around. Many have continued to take advantage of others who are less powerful than themselves. They have done so in nonsexual ways or ways that were not illegal. It seems to be a habit that is hard to break. The question of motivation to break that habit is always present.

The clinician is addressing entrenched problems in a population whose motivation develops slowly. He or she must genuinely like these individuals in order to make the challenge of confrontation and support worthwhile for him or herself. He or she must be able to see the clients' faults clearly and be able to identify with what the victims must have been feeling during their abuse. And the clinician must also see the humanity in these young people and have compassion for what their internal lives must be like to bring them to commit such acts. Anything less will make the techniques useless, for behind the techniques must be a capacity and willingness to relate to both the abuser and the hurt child in each offender.

BIBLIOGRAPHY

Benoit, Jeffrey and Kennedy, Wallace, "The Abuse History of Male Adolescent Sex Offenders," *Journal of Interpersonal Violence*, 1992, 7: 543-548.

Cunningham and MacFarlane, *When Children Molest Children*, Orwell, VT: Safer Society Press, 1991.

Dwyer, Margretta S. and Rosser, Simon B., "Treatment Outcome Research Cross-Referencing a Six Month to Ten Year Follow-up Study on Sex Offenders," *Annals of Sex Research*, 1992, 5: 87-97.

Farrenkopf, Toni, "What Happens to Therapists Who Work with Sex Offenders?" *Journal of Offender Rehabilitation*, 1992, 18: 217-223.

Freeman-Longo, Robert and Knopp, Fay H., "State-of-the-Art Sex Offender Treatment: Outcome and Issues," *Annals of Sex Research*, 1992, 5: 141-160.

Hinman, Jan, *Restitution, Treatment and Training Inc.*, Ontario, OR: Alexander Associates, 1992.

Kahn, Timothy, *Pathways: A Guided Workbook for Youth Beginning Treatment*, Orwell, VT: Safer Society Press, 1990.

Marshall, W., Laws, D.R., and Barbaree, H.E. (Eds.) *Handbook of Sexual Assault: Issues, Theories, and Treatment of the Offender*, New York: Plenum, 1989.

Mazur, Tom and Michael, P.M., "Outpatient Treatment for Adolescents with Sexually Inappropriate Behavior: Program Description and Six-Month Follow-up," *Journal of Offender Rehabilitation*, 1992, 18: 191-203.

Ryan, Gail and Lane, Sandy, *Juvenile Sexual Offending: Causes, Consequences and Correction*, Lexington, MA: Lexington Books, 1991.

Salter, Anna, *Treating Child Sex Offenders and Victims*, Newbury Park, CA: Sage Publications, 1988.

Samenow, Stanley, *Inside the Criminal Mind*, New York, NY: Random House, 1984.

Steer and Monnette, *Treating Sex Offenders in the Community*, Springfield, IL: Charles Thomas Publisher, 1989.

Wiederholt, Ingo C., "The Psychodynamics of Sex Offenses and Implications for Treatment," *Journal of Offender Rehabilitation*, 1992, 18: 19-24.

Chapter 6

Activity Group for Emotionally Disturbed Children

Mary Lou Paulsen
Kenneth F. Dunker
Joan G. Young

INTRODUCTION

The Activity Therapy Group model described was developed and is being used at the Beloit Counseling Program of Lutheran Social Service of Iowa, in Ames, Iowa. Beloit provides mental health counseling for children, adolescents, families, individuals, and couples.

The group was developed in 1973, in response to the many latency-aged children being seen who were experiencing difficulty with the growing-up process. Often this process had been interrupted or affected by abuse, parental divorce, family violence, multiple losses, parental substance abuse, attention deficit disorder, or other neurological or physiological or family problems.

The children in our groups from Central Iowa are nearly always Caucasian, but are from a varied socio-economic background. Other activity therapy groups have been used successfully with children of various racial and ethnic backgrounds, and one would also expect success with this group modality. Leaders must be prepared to discuss racial issues if they are presented just as they are ready to discuss any other issue brought up by a child. It is the therapist's role to point out issues of individuality as the children look for unity in

Portions of the text and sample forms in the appendix are reproduced from *Mastery: Making Groups Work with Children,* Second Edition, copyright © 1993, with the permission of Lutheran Social Service of Iowa.

the group. Through the group experience, children can learn that people with differences can do well together (Moss 1992, p. 100).

MODALITY DEVELOPMENT

When the group was developed, it was apparent that many latency-aged children shared common problem definitions. These were children who were not achieving in school. They lacked appropriate social skills and displayed a failure orientation and an inability to delay gratification. They had a poor self-concept and were often either overly dependent on others or inappropriately independent. It became clear that in addition to family therapy resulting in family change, the child needed to attend to some unfinished work in his or her own development. The group was developed to widen the treatment choice for children of latency age to give them an opportunity to work on early developmental tasks of latency. The group model has continued to be used successfully with six-to twelve-year-old children.

In the Beloit model, children are seen in groups because groups are a natural environment for latency-aged children. A group with peers is less threatening than individual therapy to children who have not developed trust in adults. The group experience enables children to learn social skills from each other. They can work through trust issues with adults, learn to balance independence and dependence, and further their ability to internalize inner controls.

Crafts are used as a vehicle for self-concept change. The use of crafts seems to appeal to all children. This offers a concrete way for a child to express him or herself, master his or her own skills and the tools. In addition, the completion of a craft project promotes positive feelings about the self. Crafts give children the opportunity to appreciate the productive use of time and to learn to postpone gratification.

THEORETICAL ORIENTATION

To further understand the way these groups function, we must first step back to take a closer look at the developmental tasks of the latency age child. It is well established especially through the work of Erik Erickson that as children grow they must master certain developmental tasks before moving on to the next level (Erickson 1950 and 1968). These tasks make up the foundation upon which the child builds the structure of his or her own self. Children have an inner desire to grow and to master their own bodies, their emotions, and their places within their families and play groups. The major task of latency is mastery. Mastery involves the child's ability to establish a deep, inner confidence that the self is in charge.

One may observe an infant struggling to focus on the mobile over the crib, or a one-year-old dropping blocks into a pail only to pour them out and repeat the activity. One sees a three-year-old changing clothes several times a day or a six-year-old riding a two wheel bike up and down the same block. A ten-year-old plays a new video game over and over. This is mastery. Mastery of a skill and the child's own body is a reflection of the mastery of his or her own life. At no time is mastery more significant than between the ages of six and twelve.

As with each stage of life, the tasks to be mastered during these years are numerous. These tasks include the following:

1. Developing a sense of competence and mastery
2. Enhancing a positive self-concept
3. Developing socialization skills that allow healthy relationships with peers
4. Building a commitment to his or her social community
5. Maintaining an appropriate balance between dependence and independence
6. Internalizing inner controls and ego strengths
   a. Learning to delay gratification
   b. Developing the ability for self-evaluation
   c. Accepting responsibility for one's own behavior
   d. Developing a positive attitude toward work and productivity

With successful efforts in each of these tasks, a child becomes emotionally ready to move on to the next stage of development. When these preceding tasks are not accomplished, a child's move into adolescence becomes difficult.

Many children approach life tasks (spelling tests, daily chores) expecting to fail or do poorly. Therefore, they put little effort into them, which results in failure. The group model offers a structured way to break this negative cycle. The opportunity for decision making, planning, and following a plan to completion helps children approach group tasks with a success orientation. As they enjoy the feeling of success, there is an increasing ability to generalize this experience to other areas of life. Gradually, the child begins to develop a success orientation rather than a failure orientation.

Activity therapy group does address each of the developmental tasks in several ways. Children develop competence and mastery as they learn to use tools such as saws, hammers, or the vise. As children complete their projects they feel good about themselves and their capabilities.

Self-concept improves as they learn to accept compliments about their project or the way they work. They are given the opportunity to express their likes and dislikes regarding their projects. They feel a sense of accomplishment and evaluate themselves, their skills, and their efforts positively. They begin to accept responsibility for both their mistakes and their successes.

The group gives children the opportunity, in a safe and highly structured environment, to practice new social skills. They receive feedback about the ways they relate to others. They learn to develop and maintain relationships within the group. The children begin to share feelings and experiences about themselves and their world. Members allow adults to be in charge when they realize in this setting it is safe to be a child. They recognize they are supported in their efforts to solve conflicts. Children begin to initiate positive interaction with their peers and practice new social skills.

Children begin to realize they each have an impact on the group, which eventually leads to developing a commitment to their social community. When they arrive on time, return their contract, cooperate in clean up, demonstrate positive behavior before and after the group, and set a positive example during group, it becomes apparent that they recognize this commitment. The hope is that this will generalize into the family, the classroom, and the neighborhood.

The balance between dependence and independence is a lifelong struggle. In latency, children begin to be more and more responsible for themselves. In the group, children work on this balance by asking for help only when it is needed, working on their own according to their ability. They make decisions about the project or the paint they will use or their contract. They may begin to take more initiative in the group.

Children work on developing self-control through following directions and leaving their project at the agency until it is complete. They must also listen to others, find acceptable ways to express negative feelings, and learn to handle mistakes. They learn to stay out of others' projects and problems. These challenges help children to develop their own inner control system, which is so essential for emotional happiness.

GROUP SETTING

Selection of physical space will vary from group to group. Planning available space to meet the needs of the group is more important than the actual space chosen. Use of the same space on a regular basis is important in that it provides consistency and security for both children and leaders. When children enter each group session in a familiar place, the energy that would be required in sorting out their own space can be diverted to the important task of reconnecting with peers and adult leaders. The security of knowing where you are to be and that your space is ready for you assists in a sense of belonging, in lessening of initial stress, and in stabilizing internal control systems.

A pleasant, well-lighted atmosphere communicates a sense of belonging and an invitation for enjoyment. It is also important that the space allows adults to be comfortable with the natural messiness inherent in working on projects with children. The easy availability and the organization of equipment and materials that are needed for the group's weekly activities also enable the group process to proceed smoothly. Children grow when they experience the ability to trust that adults will care for them. Their developing sense of independence is strengthened as they assume responsibility for locating what they need and maintaining their group space in an orderly manner.

GROUP GUIDELINES

Well-defined guidelines provide the basis for the structure of the group and the interactions within the group. All children need clear statements about the expectations of the group leaders and the goals of the group experience. Guidelines can and do differ. Those chosen will depend on the purpose of the group, the children involved, the personality and philosophy of the leaders, and the type of available physical space. The guidelines that are chosen need to remain constant, be made important, be clearly communicated, and be stated in positive ways. It is our experience that the group guidelines become valued by group members. The following guidelines are those used in the Beloit activity groups:

1. Caring About Others

Socializing and developing healthy peer relationships are important to the latency-aged child. Relationships are complicated by anxiety, uncertainty, and lack of experience with social skills. Most of the children referred for these groups have demonstrated significant difficulties in this area. This guideline makes this an important part of group functioning. "Caring about others" is useful in teaching children about the choices they can make in the treatment of one another. They learn how to show caring and how to deal with negative feelings. It also enables children to become more sensitive to the impact their actions and words have on their peers.

2. Following the Plan

This guideline places importance on the development of a plan to achieve a successful product. This process will enhance the child's self-concept. As children generalize this plan in other life tasks, such as a school assignment or household chores, they take a step toward approaching life tasks with a success rather than a failure orientation. It is important that the plan fit each child's ability to write.

3. Leaving Project Until Completed

One of the developmental tasks for a latency child is learning to delay gratification. This guideline can initially cause significant struggles in many children because this part of personality is in the developing stage and children are anxious to share accomplishments at home. As children grow, they begin to accept this guideline more easily. Leaders need to be very clear about defining what "completed" means–paint totally dry, fasteners attached, etc.

4. Proper Care of Tools

Children can gain skills in the way they use tools. They learn that tools work for them if they are cared for. We believe children can and do generalize from the specific tools in one environment to other tools and equipment they use in other environments. As they develop this ability, they are working on developing a personal organization. This facilitates having materials ready for a school assignment, knowing where to easily locate a favorite shirt, or remembering to put away a basketball.

5. Helping with Cleanup

This guideline helps children experience a growing adequacy and increasing independence as they learn to take personal responsibility for caring for their belongings. Each group member is also assigned one general cleanup task in the work environment. From this they gain a sense of group participation and the value of cooperative activity. Moving from work time to cleanup time is often a difficult transition. As they are able to accomplish this in group they are helped with other transitions in their lives.

6. Having Fun

This is the favorite guideline of children in the Beloit groups. It encourages an enjoyment of living whether one is spending time and energy on work or play activities, in relationship interactions, or in dealing with pleasant or difficult issues.

In our experience most children incorporate these guidelines fairly quickly, and one can frequently hear one child reminding another child of a guideline. They also occasionally test the guidelines. It is helpful and often sufficient if the primary group leader is very clear and direct about the expectation for the child. Phrasing the expectation in a positive way makes it easier for the child to accept. If adults are clear and consistent about expectation, children will understand their limits, be comfortable with them, and be more likely to accept them.

Occasionally one of the children will have difficulty in managing the group situation, causing disruption for themselves and the other group members. Within the Beloit philosophy the leader will find a way to talk with the child privately and in a warm and caring manner. Hopefully, the child can share conflicts or misunderstandings with other group members or with the group process. The leader may also gain some understanding of difficulties at school or home, that affect the child's behavior.

When a child cannot be helped within the group or individually by the leader, the problem is discussed with the parent or parents. If the parents are invested in the treatment process they will support their child's involvement in the group and communicate their expectations that guidelines be followed.

GROUP STRUCTURE

The ideal group size is five to seven members with two adult leaders and a volunteer. This is dependent on the size of the room and the availability of two leaders. From our experience, activity groups work best if there is less than a three-year range among the members. The group seems to work equally well if it is composed of all boys or all girls or a mixture of both.

The length of the group sessions can vary depending on the type of group, the planned content, and the goals of the group. After trying several time frames, the Beloit staff schedules each group session for one hour and fifteen minutes. The session begins with a fifteen-minute sharing time, continues with a forty-five minute work and cleanup time, and ends with a fifteen-minute closing time.

Sharing Time

When the group meeting begins, it is helpful to have one leader meet the group members in the reception area while the other leader waits in the group room to welcome them. It is important to begin the group on time as it encourages children to arrive on time. Establishing a traditional way to begin each meeting is a signal to get ready for group. In the Beloit model, group members greet one another with a structured "Good afternoon."

The sharing session serves a variety of functions. It is important as a "settling in" time. A child may choose to share something about his or her day or past week. The leaders, in observing the children, will gain some sense of their moods, which is helpful in assessing the kind of interactions that would be useful. Once the children feel safe in group they often share some very painful experiences. The group is amazingly caring and supportive when this happens. The leader may choose to give some direction to the sharing by suggesting a topic with a positive frame like, "Tell us something that you felt good about today."

As the sharing session ends, it helps in the transition into the work period if the leader asks each child what he or she will be doing during work time. If the child cannot remember, the child is reminded to check his or her plan.

Work Time

Children come to a group with a variety of skills, abilities, talents, and experiences. Each child needs the opportunity to focus on his or her own strengths and be allowed to feel successful. Because competition between children is to be avoided, it is important that no two children be working on the same project at any one time. The leaders will have a selected group of project possibilities, with a completed model of each, for the children to see and examine.

The first project that a child does should require only minimal handling of tools and allow for small choices for the child to make. The beginning project will assist the leader in assessing the child's skills, abilities, attention span, and frustration level. The name board works especially well for this purpose in an open-ended group. If the group is formed with all members beginning at the same time, several beginning projects should be selected.

After the first project is completed, the primary leader selects three projects from which a child can choose the one he or she wishes to make. This gives the leader some control over the project chosen in order to make it a successful experience for the child, and also defines the hierarchy of the group with the adult clearly in charge. Within these limits, the child experiences the struggles involved in decision making and gains an awareness of the factors to be considered such as the approximate length of time for completion, the difficulty level, and his or her level of interest.

The working session gives children many opportunities for growth. Positive peer interaction is more possible when competition is avoided. Children seem to be freer in offering praise and encouragement to one another. They can lend a helping hand, such as holding a board steady while it is being sawed. Again, it is important for the adult to be in charge if the children begin to offer negative comments or begin taking over another child's project.

The process of working on a project is useful in helping children find a balance between dependence and independence. Some children have difficulty in asking for or using help even when it is needed. Other children have developed a pattern of overdependence on others. Adults help by giving encouragement, making suggestions, and providing help when appropriate. The plan prepared by the child assists him or her in feeling less fearful. As the child's confidence and mastery of tasks builds, his or her independence will grow.

Mistakes will occur, and again, these provide growth experiences. Children react to mistakes in various ways. Some pretend no mistake was made. Some want to quit. Some cry or get angry. Others place blame. Growth occurs as children assume responsibility for their mistakes as well as their successes. This is learned by discovering that it is okay to make mistakes. Help is provided in correcting a mistake. It is a clear expectation that "giving up" is not an option. The sense of satisfaction and success that a child feels when a troublesome project has been completed is a joy to see.

The last few minutes of the work session are devoted to cleanup time. A warning from the leader that cleanup will be occurring helps this transition go more smoothly. Group jobs are listed on a chart and rotated weekly. When a child's cleanup is complete, the child may be encouraged to help others.

Closing Session

This is a time to share completed projects and also a time to process the group experience. A child with a completed project is asked to share the most enjoyable, the most frustrating, or the most difficult part of completing a project. In talking about the group experience group leaders let the children know what went well, which interactions they noticed, or what might have gone better. It is also a time for sharing good feelings about each other. For example, the group may go around the table giving a compliment to the person on the left. Children have difficulty in both giving and receiving compliments, and learning to do this is invaluable to a child's building a sense of self.

During the closing session, each child also develops a contract to take home. (See the example contract form in the Appendix.) The primary goal of the contract is to facilitate a feeling of competency and responsibility. It is suggested that children choose a daily task that will be of help to themselves or their families. It can be a task of showing caring by giving a parent a hug each day. It can be one that strengthens the child's sense of mastery with the daily completion of a chore. The chosen behavior can also be one that contributes to a child's sense of family, such as reading to a younger sibling.

Children are helped with the skills of choosing a goal that is achievable, measurable, and stated in positive terms. In the process of working out the contract, the child is often helped by suggestions from other group members. The child learns to listen to others as well as to get ideas and cues from others.

When the child has chosen the goal for the week, he or she completes a contract form. The contract is signed by the child and by one of the group leaders. It is the responsibility of the child to mark each day's completion of his or her goal. Before returning the contract to the group the child is asked to have a parent sign the contract.

Returned contracts are reviewed by the group with special attention given for positive efforts children have made. The group receives one point for each returned contract on which the stated goal has been accomplished on at least one day. When the group as a whole has earned a total of 15 points, the group is permitted to plan refreshments for the next week.

It is helpful if each group ends in a traditional way. It is not important exactly how the group ends, but that the ending is consistent. This builds a sense of belonging in each child as he or she becomes more comfortable and secure in knowing exactly what to expect from the group. Tradition also helps to form group cohesiveness.

Beginnings and endings are important. The beginning of each group session, just as in any beginning, may bring to each child a mixture of anxiety, fear, or excitement. It is helpful to remember that many of these children have experienced painful and frightening endings in their lives. Endings also signify beginnings. At the end of a group session, the child is thinking about going home. This creates various feelings depending on the day and on other factors. The structure of the group and traditional ways in which groups begin and end provide safety and caring, which enable a child to better cope with anxiety.

LEADERSHIP

Leaders of an activity therapy group should be trained in the treatment of children, understand children's emotional and developmental needs, and have the ability to discern how children express feelings both verbally and behaviorally. They also need to have a commitment to the goals of the group and be willing to grow themselves. Consistent involvement is critical to the group process. The leader also needs to show enthusiasm and be aware of his or her importance to the children and to the group. It is important for leaders to genuinely like children and be respectful of them as individuals. The leaders must be able to allow children to work out their feelings without interrupting or rescuing them. The leader must have a clear sense of who he or she is and not personally need the children to like him or her.

In addition, group leaders need to have an understanding of group dynamics and be able to facilitate healthy group interaction. The leader needs to trust the therapeutic process and understand that change comes in small increments. He or she needs to truly value the activity and understand how the activities relate to the children's needs. It is also important to thoroughly enjoy the value of working with one's hands so that this enjoyment can be transmitted to the children.

The most important requirement for the leader is to have good relationship ability. One must be able to support and encourage without taking over for the child. The leaders must be able to be honest with themselves and with the children, and about their own mistakes. A sense of humor always enhances one's relationship with the children.

It is best for each group to have both male and female leaders. Children identify with them and see them as role models. They also model the male-female interaction. It is also important to have leaders who represent the culture, race, and ethnicity of the children in the group.

The Beloit model has two distinct roles for leaders. These roles are not pointed out to the children, but they are very quickly understood. The primary expector is the leader who meets the children in the waiting room, leads sharing time, gives group guidelines, intervenes in conflict, and makes primary decisions. The nurturer leader assists and enables the children to meet expectations and to feel successful. A volunteer or student is frequently used as a third leader. Three leaders give children more personalities to model, and it is useful to have three adults observing group interaction.

PROJECTS

Concept, Selection, and Examples

The project shelf and ceiling in the Beloit activity group room presently contain more than 70 project models. The number of models has grown from 10 to 15 as the original set has been supplemented periodically.

For each of the projects, the concept is to move from plan development to project completion using basic materials. Each project begins when a child copies a model plan from either the wood or non-wood project notebook. (See the name board plan in the Appendix.) With group leader permission, the child may modify the plan but once the plan is completed the child is expected to follow that plan until the project is complete.

Using basic materials carries the risk of failure. Children make mistakes selecting materials, measuring and cutting parts, assembling parts, and painting. It is important that activity group leaders be prepared to deal with these mistakes. In general there are two choices to remedy mistakes: (1) remake the part or (2) adapt the mistake as a special feature within the general limits of the plan.

As an example of working with a mistake, consider a string art project that involves a ring of nails to be strung with a five-pointed star. A child accidentally overlapped the two parts of the nail pattern in such a way that the ring of nails had two fewer than required. Because of the child's treatment schedule and her investment in pounding in the nails, a group leader gave her the option of stringing the nails with a series of rings rather than the star. Her pattern was different than the project model but within the plan task of "string yarn around nails."

Projects are selected for use in the group on the basis of several criteria. A project must depend on easily learned skills because children come to the group with a variety of skills and lack of skills. Some children will try to fake a skill, and group leaders need to be alert to the needs of a new child in group. If skills for a project are not easy to learn, a group leader will need to work exclusively with one child and will be unable to work with other children or to deal effectively with group interaction issues.

Any project for use in the group needs to be divisible into a series of small tasks. These tasks then can be used by the group leaders for planning immediately before the group begins. Additionally, the list of tasks gives a child a structure for working on the project and, to indicate progress, the tasks may be checked off when completed.

A project should be based on simple materials, otherwise ordering and purchasing can be difficult. A long lead time in obtaining a key material, if forgotten, can turn a child's project into a very frustrating experience. Even simple materials can pose problems, however. Many of the small projects with wheels used at Beloit were planned for large macrame beads. When the beads became unavailable, plastic toilet seat washers were a substitute. At this time, mail-order wooden model wheels often are the only alternative. A group leader must plan ahead for projects with wheels because a last-minute run to a local store is not an option.

A variety of projects interesting to children is an important drawing card for an activity group. Often a Beloit staff member can overcome a child's resistance to beginning the activity group treatment simply by showing the child the project shelf. The process of starting with a plan and basic materials and working to completion builds a sense of accomplishment. Projects should be selected for the project shelf with an eye toward the sense of satisfaction children can achieve.

Many of the children want power tools to complete projects at a faster pace. For safety reasons, in addition to treatment considerations, projects need to be constructed without power tools. Relatively dangerous hand tools such as chisels or knives also need to be excluded. Safety is important because a group leader cannot be with every child all of the time. Eye protection and other appropriate safety equipment must be available and prescribed by a group leader, if necessary.

Creativity is a consideration when selecting projects. Kits and excessive use of prefabricated materials remove creativity from projects, and the construction process becomes an assembly line operation. Kits remove many of the opportunities for frustration with projects and the associated opportunities of dealing with a child's treatment issues.

Because children come to group with a variety of skills and develop skills during the group process, it is important to select projects at different levels of skill and difficulty. Projects in use at Beloit provide for graded levels of skill and require anywhere from one week to three months to complete. Group leaders have the responsibility of helping a child select a project to meet an appropriate skill level and time commitment.

Ten example projects—name board, puzzle game, bookends, teddy bear, marionette, string art, bulletin board, bird feeder, catamaran, and train—are described in detail in Part II of *Mastery* (Paulsen, Dunker, and Young, 1993, pp. 74-164). In the order listed above, the projects require increasing levels of skill and increasing time commitments.

The name board, the first project that all children make when they enter activity group, introduces the child to group and indirectly provides a name tag for several weeks. Although some group leaders may choose to have a child start the name board from scratch, the authors generally have prepared the board with the child's name in advance. The prepared board is set out with the model plan when the new child enters the room for the first group session so that the child has a head start on the project. The new child's project is part of the group's partially completed projects.

Skills required for the name board are minimal. Often the child will customize his or her name in a way reflecting personality or treatment issues.

At the end of the list are the relatively difficult projects that children complete near the end of their time in activity group. For relatively skilled children, those projects–bird feeder, catamaran, or train–become masterpiece projects that demonstrate their mastery of group treatment objectives. For less skilled children, marionette or string art projects may serve as appropriate masterpiece projects.

Room Setup

As noted above, an activity group program requires some commitment for physical space and inventory of materials. Present facilities at Beloit are a 15-foot by 17-foot group room and a 15-foot by 7-foot materials room, with a supplemental materials storage closet below a stair. Those facilities are comfortable for a group of five to seven children with leaders and have served four or five treatment groups regularly scheduled during a week. A single room of about half the size of the present group room, with supplemental materials storage, was tight but adequate for a group of four children and two leaders. Although the group room must be set up for craft projects, it also may be used for other types of treatment sessions and for small staff meetings.

Within the activity group room there should be a bulletin board area for each group. Group leaders may choose to establish a theme for the group, such as Tuesday zoo, California Raisins, or Garfield Street. With a theme, each child and group leader can be given a paper cutout on the bulletin board, and the cutouts can be coordinated with a cleanup chart. Also, the bulletin board should have a tally sheet for returned contracts and an envelope for those contracts. Children are expected to place their contracts in the envelope and post their points as they enter the group room. The group's bulletin board also serves as a collection point for the active project plans.

Also within the activity room there is need for appropriate furniture. Group guidelines should be prominently posted near a sharing table. Although the sharing table and chairs may be sized for adults, the other items of furniture–the project table and workbench–should have lower work surfaces appropriate for children in the group. The sharing table and chairs should accommodate the maximum number of children and group leaders. In addition, it may be appropriate to have an extra time-out chair in the room or hallway.

Somewhere in the room should be a leaders' corner with both accessible and out-of-reach shelves and drawers. At the child-accessible levels, project plans and patterns, paper supplies, and completed projects ready for sharing can be stored. At the upper levels, group leaders can keep personal items and other items such as the cleanup bell to end work time.

An attractive display of the model projects is made possible with a project shelf along a wall of the group room. Models should be accessible to the children because a model of the child's project often will answer questions about construction and procedure. When a child is in the process of choosing the next project, a group leader can place several project models on a table as a focus for the choice.

Items such as materials and tools that may be distractions during sharing time may be stored in a separate materials room. The material storage should include a lumber rack, a paint locker (or suitable storage required by the local fire inspector), nail and small-parts cabinets, and storage racks for containers of larger, loose materials. A pegboard at child-accessible level with hooks locked in place generally provides tool storage so that children can see and reach the necessary tools.

There needs to be storage for partially completed projects, perhaps in a cabinet. Freshly painted or glued projects, however, should have separate, open storage. Within the material storage room is the best place for the sink and cleanup tools such as brooms, brushes, and dustpans. The separate materials room has both the advantage that distractions are out of sight and the disadvantage that a child can get lost among the distractions when group leaders are not alert.

Group Procedures

After the child's first project–the name board–the child should be given some choice for subsequent projects. Usual procedure with the Beloit groups is to give the child three choices, of which one may be the child's choice. At the time the child chooses the next project, the group leader needs to consider the child's ability as well as treatment objectives and communicate the considerations with the choices. Materials and supplies also may be a consideration.

Once the child has made the choice, he or she has permission to find the model plan in the appropriate notebook and copy the plan. The child should add his or her name to the plan and request permission from a group leader for any changes to the model plan. For various reasons, it is a good idea to require that a group leader check a child's plan before proceeding.

In general, a plan should have specific tasks sequenced as follows: mark, cut and drill, shape and prepare, finish, and assemble. The finish and assemble tasks may be interchanged depending on the complexity of the finishes. As a child progresses through a project, the sequence may need to be modified to fit available time during a group session. A child, however, should not need to modify the sequence because of lack of materials or tools. The group leader needs to check supplies at the time of the project choice if there is any availability question.

Sharing a completed project should be a happy time for the child. Sharing is planned for the closing group session, after contracts for the next week are completed by all. Each child and group leader is expected to give at least one compliment. A good question with which to close the project sharing is, "What will you do with the project?" A child's investment in the treatment group, progress, and relationship with his or her family often are evident in the answer.

ASSESSMENT

This activity group model has been developed to provide growth and change opportunities for each child. Very specifically defined and articulated goals are of primary importance in several ways.

1. They define the basis for the structure and format of a group. Decisions about group leadership, planned activities, length of group meetings, physical space requirements, and guidelines are made in relationship to stated goals.
2. They define the membership of the group. Goals are selected and defined to meet the needs of a potential group of children who exhibit similar needs. Those children whose needs can be met through group participation are easily defined.

3. The goals provide a measuring stick for the weekly process of the group interactions and activities. They become tools for leaders to assess group climate, leadership functioning, and project assessment.
4. Most importantly, they chart the progress for each child. This information is used in tailoring the child's participation to help the child move toward realization of his or her goals. Through awareness of the goals on which he or she is working, the child can also learn to self-evaluate progress. The child will understand what he or she needs to accomplish before graduation. Most children can articulate the changes that they have made at that time. The child's progress is also shared with his or her parents as part of the overall family treatment process. They are encouraged to support the goals their child is working toward and to incorporate the intent of the goals into the home environment.

The activity group model advocated in this chapter addresses the needs of the latency-aged child and especially the child who is experiencing difficulties in moving through his or her developmental tasks. Thus, the goals of these groups are focused on these tasks. Six specific goals are used. Each goal is defined with measurable objectives.

A child's progress is measured and recorded in two ways. The first is a weekly progress review. (See the sample weekly progress review in the Appendix.) After each group session, the team of group leaders completes a review for each child, defining his or her strengths as well as struggles. Ongoing work with each child is based on the reviews. They are also shared with the family therapist to provide information and to facilitate family work.

The second progress measurement is a 90-day review. (See the sample 90-day review form in the appendix.) In the Beloit program, it is the responsibility of the primary therapist to communicate with parents about their child's participation in group. The 90-day review completed by the group leadership team assists this process.

Recognizing that change occurs slowly over a period of time, this review presents a broader picture of a child's progress. This encourages parents to validate the growth in their child. It also becomes an additional tool in the work they are doing to make systemic changes in the family.

Having worked with hundreds of children using this group modality, it has been rare to find a child who has not shown growth in his or her goals. With a strong investment in the treatment process by the parent or parents, change might occur more rapidly. Without significant change in the family system, we have experienced that many children demonstrate growth in ego strength and relationship ability. This model of group therapy does enable developmental gains leading to better preparation for adolescent years.

APPENDIX
Name Board Plan

NAME BOARD

MATERIALS

- 1 × 4 board
- beans, corn, macaroni
- yarn
- glue
- stain
- varnish

DIRECTIONS

1. Sand board.*
2. Drill holes.
3. Stain board.
4. Glue beans, corn, or macaroni.
5. Varnish.
6. Thread yarn through holes.
7. Cut and tie yarn.

---

* This plan assumes that a group leader has cut the name board and stenciled on the child's name in advance.

Activity Group Contract Form

ACTIVITY GROUP CONTRACT   Date _____

I have agreed to work on _____

during this next week.

Wednesday   _____

Thursday   _____

Friday   _____

Saturday   _____

Sunday   _____

Monday   _____

Tuesday   _____

Signed:

Child   _____

Therapist   _____

Parent   _____

I will return this at the next group meeting.

Weekly Activity Group
Progress Review Form

Case Name _____   Providers _____

Date _____ Rating Scale: 1   2   3   4   5
                                     positive   needs improvement

Commitment to Group:

____ Here on time   ____ Returns contract   ____ Cooperates in
                                                               clean-up

____ Ends on time   ____ Respectful behavior
                                before and after group

Competency and Mastery:

____ Proper use of tools   ____ Attends to project
                                and follows plan

____ Demonstrates a
     sense of accomplishment

Balance Between Dependence/Independence:

____ Asks for help   ____ Follows through on
     when needed   instructions

Acquired Social Skills and Self-Control:

____ Uses feedback to   ____ Listens to others and
     modify behavior   shares about self

____ Initiates positive   ____ Allows adults to
     interaction with   be in charge
     others

Improved Self-Concept

____ Accepts compliments   ____ Expresses feelings
                                constructively

____ Appropriately
     expresses likes and
     dislikes

Level of Participation: over   expected   under

Other Impressions:

Signature _____

Ninety-Day Progress
Review Form

ACTIVITY GROUP GOALS: 90-DAY REVIEW

Case Name _____   Group _____

Date _____   Completed by _____

Goal 1. Develop a sense of competence and mastery as demonstrated
by ability to complete a range of projects successfully.

Goal 2. Develop an improved self-concept as demonstrated by
broadening awareness of and gaining acceptance of own
strengths and limitations.

Goal 3. Learn and practice social skills appropriate for his or her
age by developing positive relationships with adult
and peers.

Goal 4. Experience building a commitment to his or her social community as demonstrated by his or her ongoing investment in and contribution to the group process.

Goal 5. Achieve a balance of dependence and independence as demonstrated by ability to be appropriately self-rUliant and to trust others for help when needed.

Goal 6. Learn and practice self-control as demonstrated by ability to attend to tasks, to channel feelings of frustration, and to share time and attention with others.

REFERENCES

Erickson, Erik. 1950. *Childhood and society.* New York: Norton Press.
————. 1968. *Identity, youth and crisis.* New York: Norton Press.
Moss, Wendy. 1992. Group psychotherapy with adolescents in a residential treatment center. *Journal of Child and Adolescent Group Therapy,* 2(2): 93-104.
Paulsen, M. L., K. F. Dunker, and J. Young. 1993. *Mastery: Making groups work with children, second edition.* Ames: Lutheran Social Service of Iowa.

BIBLIOGRAPHY

Baughman, Glenn. 1973. Crafts and commitment: A supportive treatment experience for disturbed children. Unpublished paper, Child Guidance Center, Des Moines, IA.
Coyle, Grace Longwell. 1948. *Group work with American youth: A guide to the practice of leadership.* New York: Harper and Brothers Publishers.
Friberg, Selma H. 1959. *The magic years.* New York: Charles Scribner's Sons.
Ginott, Haim G. 1961. *Group psychotherapy with children: The theory and practice of play-therapy.* New York: McGraw-Hill Book Co., Inc.
Jones, Mary Nel. 1973. A systems approach to latency age activity groups for emotionally disturbed children. Master's thesis, School of Social Work, University of Iowa, Iowa City, IA.
Konopka, Gisela. 1949. *Therapeutic group work with children.* Minneapolis, MN: University of Minnesota Press.
Roos, Barbara Madej, and Shirley Armintrout Jones. 1982. Working with girls experiencing loss: An application of activity group therapy in a multiethnic community. *Social Work with Groups,* 5 (Fall):35-49.
Sarroff, Charles. 1976. *Latency.* New York: Jason Aronson, Inc.

Chapter 7

Multiple-Family Therapy Groups: A Responsive Intervention Model for Inner-City Families

Mary McKernan McKay
J. Jude Gonzales
Susan Stone
David Ryland
Katherine Kohner

Having parents and their children meet together to share information, address common concerns, or develop supportive networks
can be an efficient and effective means of providing child and
family mental health services. This chapter will provide a clinical
description of a multiple-family therapy group (MFTG) developed
to meet the needs of inner-city children and their families at an
urban child mental health center. The development of responsive
intervention modalities for low-income minority children and families is critical given their increased risk for psychopathology. Yet,
there are clear indications that this vulnerable client population is
less likely to be met by responsive service providers and relevant
intervention modalities (Kazdin, 1993; Tuma, 1989; Brandenburg
et al., 1987; Cheung and Snowden, 1989; Flaskerud, 1986; Gary,
1982; Sue, 1977). MFTGs offer the opportunity to decrease the
stigma associated with mental health services and increase engagement of "at-risk" children and families (Aponte et al., 1991; Boyd-
Franklin, 1993). In this chapter, multiple family therapy groups will
be defined and a brief literature review of their past uses and clinical benefits will be presented. A model for how MFTGs can address

child behavioral difficulties will be outlined. Goals and format of these groups will be discussed. The structure and process by which these groups address the needs of inner-city children and families will be discussed. Case examples will highlight the opportunities for change that the group provides. Obstacles that group facilitators must confront will also be identified.

MFTGs have tended to lack definitional clarity. Practioners have defined them as having widely different formats and membership criteria. O'Shea and Phelps (1985) define multiple-family groups in the most recent review of the literature related to this treatment modality to date. An MFTG has been referred to as

> . . . a deliberate, planful, psychosocial intervention with two or more families present in the same room with a trained therapist for all or most of the sessions. Each participating family should have two or more members that represent at least two generations in the family and are present for all or most of the sessions. Sessions should have an explicit focus on problems or concerns shared by all families in attendance. These focal problems should pertain directly or indirectly to cross-generational family interaction. Sessions should implicitly or explicitly emphasize patterns of interfamilial interaction, as well as utilize actual or potential alliances among members of different families based on similarities of age, sex, focal problem, or family role. (p. 555)

This rather lengthy description can be summarized with three major points: (1) these groups include children, parents, and a facilitator; (2) these groups are problem-focused; and (3) these groups are explicitly interactionally oriented, both within family unit interaction and between family interactions. Within the literature, there are several cases where multiple-family groups included only parents or where families were divided, usually along generational lines, for substantial portions of the group. A common example would be where parents meet to discuss parenting issues and children meet to play or discuss issues among themselves. These would not be considered MFTGs for the purposes of this article. Although separation of children and parents may occur as part of an activity in the group to be described, the focus of the group is primarily on children and parents participating together for the majority of the time spent in group.

These multiple-family groups are currently being developed and implemented at the Institute for Juvenile Research (IJR), the Child Psychiatry Division of the University of Illinois at Chicago. IJR is an inner-city, child mental health agency, with 67 percent of the children living with their mothers in single-parent households and an additional 21.3 percent residing with a single, female relative, such as a grandmother or aunt. Approximately 85 percent of the 450 families who requested services last year were supported by Public Assistance. Almost two-thirds of children seen at the agency are African American, 12 percent are Hispanic, and the remaining portion are White. Only brief references to the use of MFTGs with urban families can be found within the literature.

REVIEW OF MULTIPLE-FAMILY GROUP LITERATURE

Specific attention to the use of MFTGs for treatment overall is still relatively infrequent. References to their use can be found within both the family therapy and group treatment literatures. There have been two review articles that integrate the existing work related to MFTGs (O'Shea and Phelps, 1985; Strenlick, 1978). MFTGs have been primarily incorporated within inpatient psychiatric settings with schizophrenic adults (e.g., O'Shea et al., 1991; Anderson, 1986; Laqueur, 1980; Curry, 1965). There are far fewer references to the use of MFTGs in inpatient psychiatric settings with children and adolescents (e.g., Kadis and McClendon, 1981; Reiss and Costell, 1977).

Multiple-family therapy groups have received support from clinicians working with children and adolescents in outpatient settings (Leichter and Schulman, 1986; Leichter and Schulman, 1972; Cassano, 1989a; Szymanski and Kiernan, 1983; Libo et al., 1971). In addition, MFTGs are often recommended as a potentially effective treatment modality with "multiproblem" families (Aponte et al., 1991; Leichter and Schulman, 1981), African-American families (Boyd-Franklin, 1993; Foley, 1982), and with battered women and their children (Rhodes and Zelman, 1986).

On a theoretical level, Lacqueur (1980, 1976), is most clearly linked with the development of MFTGs and the definition of their essential clinical elements. MFTGs are described as creating competition among families, thus stimulating change more quickly than might otherwise occur. Change is achieved by identification with other families "who have been there." In addition, multiple-family therapy groups allow families to practice new behaviors in a protective, supportive environment. In fact, the presence of other families can be more powerful than the therapist by providing motivation and encouragement for change. The feedback of other families can be less threatening than suggestions offered by the therapists.

Although there is clinical support for multiple-family therapy groups, empirical evidence remains limited. Five outcome studies and two observational studies were completed prior to the 1985 review article (Gould and Glick, 1977; Anton et al., 1981; Falloon, et al., 1981; Falloon and Liberman, 1983; Hardcastle, 1977; Reiss and Costell, 1977; Gould and DeGroot, 1981). Supportive findings include Hardcastle's (1977) study of mothers and their latency-age children referred because they were exhibiting behavior problems at school. Those who attended an MFTG reported decreased negative behavior by their mothers in comparison to a no-treatment control group. Empirical support for the effectiveness of multiple-family therapy groups has been hampered by study limitations, most notably that MFTGs are only one component of a treatment package offered to a family and non-equivalence between treatment and comparison groups, small sample size, and other methodological flaws exist (O'Shea and Phelps, 1985).

DESCRIPTION OF THERAPEUTIC
CHANGE PROCESS

Therapeutic work within the multiple family group being developed at IJR is guided by a family systems perspective (Tolan, Florsheim, McKay, and Kohner, 1993; Breunlin, Schwartz, and Karrer, 1993). From this perspective, the large group is viewed as a functioning system, with each individual member and family unit serving a particular role and purpose. Interactions between families are viewed as opportunities to obtain information and feedback in order to bring about change within individual family units. Change within families is precipitated through the process of presenting themselves as families to others. An individual familys' child management practices, organization, and beliefs become the focus of discussion within the larger group as well as being evaluated within the family. Furthermore, the practice portion of each group attempts to bring about family change, which then has an effect on the larger group. Children's behavior is viewed as being altered by shifts in the relationship that they have with parents, brought about by both interactions with other families and the development of more positive family interactional patterns. The theoretical model in Figure 7.1 attempts to highlight the process of change that guided the development of the multiple-family group.

The progression of clinical work within MFTGs has been discussed as consisting of sequential phases: a beginning, middle, and ending phase. Decisions as to the inclusion of members mark the *beginning of the first phase* of treatment. Criteria for inclusion include those families that can benefit from education around a particular problem. Families that need to address social isolation, division of family role responsibilities, or lifestyle transitions should be considered for multiple family therapy groups (Cassano, 1989a).

For this particular group, families were recruited through their primary therapists. It was open to families with at least one school-age child. All family members and significant relatives/others in the household were invited to attend. Families with extreme safety concerns (e.g., current child abuse/neglect or active suicidal ideation) were excluded. Caretakers presented a range of concerns about their children prior to beginning the group. The majority of the children were experiencing behavioral problems both at home and at school. In all cases, parents identified themselves as overwhelmed by these behavioral difficulties and in need of support.

Generally, groups range in size from 10 to 22 members. It was found that four to five families is the ideal size for a group. Children can range in age from preschool to adolescent. Presented difficulties are generally not identical. For example, within an ongoing group, two of the following families are present. The first family consists of a single, Mexican-American mother of three boys ranging in age

FIGURE 7.1. Multiple-Family Therapy Groups Change Process

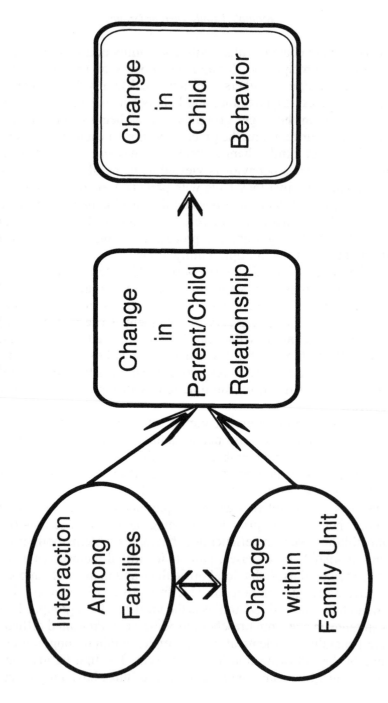

McKay, M., Gonzales, J., Stone, S., and Ryland, D. (1994).

from 10 to 17 years. She initially approached the agency for assistance with her youngest son, who was fighting on the bus to school, stealing, and lying. However, upon joining the group, she also identified difficulty with the older boys, particularly around the completion of chores and aggressive conflicts with each other. This mother was quite isolated. All of her family continued to live in Mexico. She described herself as not being successful in developing friendships in this country.

Within the same group, a 72-year-old, African-American grandmother brought her two school-age grandchildren. She had cared for the children since their births, as their mother was a substance abuser. The oldest child, a boy, was having considerable difficulty coming directly home from school. He would also leave the family home without informing his grandmother and had been picked up by the police for throwing rocks at cars on two occasions. He and his sister fought aggressively. The grandmother expressed confusion as to why her attempts to enforce rules were not effective.

Even though the family situations might appear to be quite different, the connection between these two families is impressively strong. This connection is fostered during the *beginning phase* of the group, in that families are encouraged to share their goals with other families. The process of development of group norms helps to build cohesiveness of the group. Rearing children in an urban environment, perceived as extremely dangerous to both parents and children, often brings families together during the beginning stage of the group. Gangs and pervasive drug use are commonly expressed concerns. The consequences of children making mistakes and not following rules set out to protect them often are issues that begin to connect families early in this group.

As the group progresses to its *middle phase*, members increasingly look to their peers for input. Members serve to support, confront, and lend problem-solving abilities to their peers. Members gradually refer to the multiple-family therapy groups as "our group" (Cassano, 1989a). It is during this middle phase that issues of both class and racial/ethnic differences between the families themselves and between the members and the facilitators are raised. For example, the mother and grandmother described above used corporal punishment extensively with the children. However, within the same group, there was another African-American mother who viewed physical discipline as unacceptable. Both African-American families articulated their struggles around what methods of discipline are sanctioned by their racial community. They also questioned whether other group members or the facilitators could understand the elements of racism and oppression that contributed to their views of rearing their children.

Given that members can heavily invest in the treatment process, as well as in their relationships with other members, responses to the *ending phase* of the group can be intense. Sessions devoted to evaluating experiences in the group are critical. The last group meeting also is structured as a focus group to allow the families to have input into the format of the next group series.

DESCRIPTION OF THE GROUP

The multiple-family group developed at IJR was modeled from a delinquency prevention study that utilized multiple-family groups as part of its family intervention component (Guerra, Huessmann, Tolan, VanAcker, and Eron, 1990; Tolan, Florsheim, McKay, and Kohner, 1993). Groups are held on a weekly basis for 90 minutes and co-facilitated by a male and female therapist. The groups are structured into five parts. Each group begins with an opportunity for the families to reconnect with each other and to provide updates about issues that impacted their respective family since the previous group meeting. Then, the workers facilitate the information portion of the meeting, which usually consumes 20 to 30 minutes of the total session. The remainder of the time is divided equally between group discussion, family practice exercises, and explanation of homework task (Tolan, Florsheim, McKay, and Kohner, 1993). Topics covered during the pilot eight-week group are as follows.

Week 1

Parents are asked to introduce themselves and their children. The facilitators provide a brief overview of the topics that will be discussed over the next eight weeks. Then, families are asked to identify the key ingredients of a strong family. Responses are applied to topics that will be covered in later weeks. Shared concerns among families are highlighted by the facilitators. Goals for this first session include (1) helping families identify the group as relevant to their concerns, (2) having each group member speak at least once during the session, and (3) assisting families in identifying goals for future work within the group.

Week 2

The second session focuses on the identification of family strengths, which are described as the "building blocks" for goal achievement. Identification of strengths within both mothers and their children is critical. Specific aims for this session include (1) reframing the role of child and parent as being competence-based, (2) creating a context for more positive interactional patterns between children and parents, and (3) helping group members connect within a positive, potentially less threatening format.

Weeks 3 and 4

The next two sessions focus on the development of a set of functional family rules. The need for rules to be specific, age appropriate, and consistently applied is discussed (Patterson and Forgath, 1987). Reasonable rewards and consequences become integrated into the set of family rules. Families are asked to identify rules that are more or less easily enforced. The help of other group members is actively sought. Differences between family expectations for children, level of involvement between mother and child, and comfort with corporal punishment generally emerge during these sessions. Facilitators continue to identify common themes between families. However, group members are also more likely to respond directly to each other. Group facilitators allow members to struggle with tension and difference in an effort to clarify positions and values, along with creating conditions for change.

Goals for the third and fourth session include: (1) members exchanging more with each other and less with group facilitators, (2) members having the opportunity to examine the organizational structure within the family, (3) members having exposure to information regarding effective parenting strategies, (4) members being challenged to address rules that are not being followed or easily enforced, and (5) options for rewards and consequences being explored.

Weeks 5 and 6

The next two group sessions focus on strengthening communication between adults and children within the family. Adults are described as being the "communication role models" for their children. Therefore, a strong emphasis is placed upon parents listening to, rather than talking to (or in many instances, lecturing), their children. Information regarding effective listening skills is discussed. Skills for encouraging communication among others are modeled by the facilitators and group members. Members are asked to "catch" each other when they have communicated effectively with each other or their children and give positive feedback.

Goals for these sessions include: (1) members continuing to give more feedback to each other directly, (2) members having the opportunity to practice new skills and receive reinforcement, (3) members being challenged when communication breaks down or becomes one-way in the group, and (4) children having the experience of being listened to by their caretakers.

Week 7

The last informational session focuses on managing stress related to parenting and the environment. Barriers to implementing the previously discussed topics are identified by members. An active problem-solving approach is used to think about these obstacles. Families provide support to each other and give practical suggestions. Themes of poverty, limited money, food, and parental energy are common within this session. Issues within the environment, particularly safety, substandard housing, and discrimination, are often discussed.

Goals for this session include (1) members taking responsibility as "experts" within their environment; (2) providing opportunities for members to directly identify the barriers to implementation of new parenting or relationship strategies; (3) members providing support, understanding, and encouragement for each other; and (4) members identifying and validating the existence of harmful environmental factors is validated.

Week 8

During the last group session, goals for beyond the group are set. Again, obstacles and resources within and outside the family are tied with the possibility for goal attainment. This session is facilitated as a focus group in order to get feedback for improving future groups. Members are asked to identify both positive and negative aspects of participation. Negative comments generally need to be actively solicited, with the facilitators helping to identify points where the group struggled. In the case of the current MFTGs, members were offered the possibility of continuing the group for another eight sessions. All members chose to continue with the group.

Goals for the last group session include (1) summarizing the themes of the group, (2) identifying if families have actually made changes within their families, (3) clarifying how these changes will remain in place, and (4) problem solving around inevitable obstacles for maintenance and further change.

PROCESS OF FACILITATION

Rather than giving information in a lecture format, a set of specific questions related to the topics are asked of both parents and children. Responses from group members are compiled to develop a cohesive set of principles that can then be implemented by the families. For example, during weeks 3 and 4, both parents and children are asked to identify rules in their household. Then, facilitators encourage group members to identify those rules that are being followed and those that are not. Ideas regarding the essential elements for effective rules, such as specificity, age appropriateness, and clarity are highlighted from the responses of the members. The discussion is then summarized for members so that this new knowledge can be applied to the next portion of the group session.

The next portion of the session focuses on family practice exercises. For example, the group is asked to break into individual family units to identify rules that are not followed. The group facilitators move among individual family units to encourage discussion and provide positive feedback. Other examples of family practice exercises include one family role-playing a common disagreement with the other families offering suggestions that might have been previously untried.

Finally, a relevant homework task is introduced. For example, parents might be asked to have a discussion with their children regarding a topic that emerged within the session.

Clinical Strengths of Multiple-Family Therapy Groups

1. Building Support for Parenting

Multiple-family therapy groups provide necessary conditions from which social support can be built. First, participation can validate a parent's personal experience of parenting as a stressful enterprise. In particular, the role of a single mother with limited financial resources, within the inner city is often accompanied by feelings of depression and uncertainty as to whether her efforts will be sufficient enough to protect her children from the "pulls of the street."

Over the course of the current group, parents within the group began to discuss the fears they had about their children getting into trouble, particularly in relation to joining a gang or using drugs. Many parents compared their childhood experience to that of their children and concluded that their children are growing up under circumstances that are significantly more dangerous than those they had experienced. The group facilitators raised the importance of a parent's role in relation to monitoring the whereabouts of children and setting limits that address safety. As single mothers, each questioned whether they had sufficient energy and authority to fulfill these parental functions. The group members problem-solved around who could assist them in these parenting tasks. In addition, portions of the group meetings were spent exploring how a clear family organizational structure, with age-appropriate expectations for children, could lesson the stress of single parenthood.

Participation in an MFTG can also provide the opportunity to decrease overall social isolation. Several of the group members described themselves as estranged from their own extended families. Overall, mothers reported small social networks and often included children as a major source of support. Several mothers described the group as "the only chance I get to talk to other adults."

2. Exposure to New Parenting Skills

During the didactic portion of each group, parents were presented information about the previously outlined topics. Other group members provided equally valuable suggestions around how to parent children. More important, other parents offered step-by-step advice about how to implement new ideas into the family structure. In fact, as the group progressed, members took the lead in having other members practice skills. On one occasion, a parent encouraged another parent to give her child the clear message that she was in charge of the household by saying, "Repeat after me, I am the mother. You (the child) must follow the rules because they will keep you safe." In another instance, a mother shared with the group her system of conveying rules and expectations for her children through a set of signs she had made with her children.

The extent to which families participate in the group process is not always a clear indication of the usefulness of the group to the family. For example, within the group, a mother of three children rarely spoke during the meetings. Even when actively engaged by the therapist or other parents, her answers were often brief and her manner somewhat embarrassed. However, during individual meetings with the worker following the groups, she would describe her attempts to actively incorporate the other parents' methods of discipline or communication techniques. At the end of the program, she acknowledged the development of more effective family rules, including her incorporation of another familys' suggestion that children not be allowed to watch television until they have completed their homework and household chores. She emphasized, "I never thought my kids would go along with me, until I heard Mrs. B. say that she is in charge of her house so she decides when the television goes on, not her children."

3. Multiple Sources of Feedback on Parenting

At times, feedback from other group members is more easily accepted than it might be from the therapist. For example, a mother of three was being battered by her husband. She chose one of the last groups of the program to share this with the other families. Another member in the group responded immediately and emphasized that she did not deserve to be treated violently. In discussing her decision to seek shelter later that week, she referred to the parent's comments as being an influential factor as she sought help.

Other families often can reinforce skills that might be difficult for a particular family to incorporate. For example, one single mother experienced much difficulty helping her school-age children remain in the group room or pay attention to the discussion. Over the course of the pilot, other parents in the group served a variety of roles in relation to this problem. At times, they would actively support her efforts and remind the children directly to listen to their mother's directions. At other times, they would offer her new techniques to encourage cooperation from the children. They served to remind her when she was not monitoring her children and enthusiastically complimented her when she was effective.

4. Racial/SES/Power Differences Between Therapist and Client Can Be Less of a Barrier to Participation in Treatment

The psychotherapy literature clearly indicates that a significant barrier to the engagement and retention of poor, African-American families in treatment is the frequent disparity between family and therapist in relation to race and class differences (Sue, 1977; Acosta, 1980). One of the most critical aspects of MFTGs is the reliance on other group members. This relies on traditions of self-help, mutual support, and reliance on more informal networks for help, often considered crucial in providing service to the African-American community (Boyd-Franklin, 1993). Within the pilot group, families described feeling particularly understood since other members "had been there."

In relation to the power imbalance between families and therapists, it must be acknowledged that the facilitators bring expertise to the group setting in the form of knowledge regarding parenting and skills for creating an atmosphere that maximizes the strengths of members and ensures safety and respect. As the group progresses, the therapist much less actively directs interaction between members. The group more spontaneously discusses topics and encourages practice among the members. Parents come to view themselves as having expertise, rather than relying on the therapists as "experts."

5. Opportunities for Children to Listen to Parents and Parents to Hear Children in an Alternate Context

During focus-group sessions, several parents commented that the group provided a chance to intensely focus on their children. They described themselves as being surprised by the insights and suggestions that their children offered during the group. They also mentioned an increased feeling of closeness to their children in the group as they represented their family to others in the group.

6. Opportunities to Practice Skills as a Family

A significant portion of the group is spent in practice exercise geared toward helping families experiment with new behavior. Some examples of practice exercises include having parents and children develop rules together and present to the group for feedback; interviewing each other regarding the events of the day; and giving each other information regarding important topics, such as gang activity in their neighborhoods.

While multiple-family groups can be beneficial to parents and children, they are not without challenges to group facilitators. More specifically, convening a multiple-family group means engaging diverse families around similar issues. In addition, it means addressing members from divergent developmental levels. How the complexity of the processes is managed is critical to whether discussions and practice exercises are productive for members.

Challenges to Group Facilitators

1. Parents Could Be Influenced Negatively Without Skillful Group Facilitation

Group facilitators actively define parents as having strengths and expertise in relation to their children. Many of the group members, however, have their own history of inconsistent or abusive parenting. Many group members rely on harsh parenting methods, particularly corporal punishment, to ensure cooperation by their children. During the group, reframing is used to identify a parent's goal to enhance a child's cooperation or learning. The challenge to group facilitators is to clearly identify some suggestions offered as not useful to others, while not discouraging future participation. Group facilitators have been more confident in later weeks that parents will respond by encouraging other parents to reconsider their current techniques. In contrast, during the beginning weeks of the group, the facilitators have relied upon the process of helping a parent explore the effectiveness and appropriateness of harsh strategies.

2. Group Must Address Diverse Developmental Levels

One of multiple-family group's greatest strengths relates to the simultaneous involvement of parents and their children. Yet, addressing the needs of children along with their parents is also one of the greatest challenges to facilitators. Therefore, specific questions for both parents and children related to the topic are prepared prior to group meetings. In addition, one of the goals for the first and second group is to define developmentally appropriate behavior for the children. The facilitators in collaboration with parents identify how long children should be expected to attend to discussion, sit in their seats, etc. As part of that process, members decide how the behavior of children will be addressed. For example, children under five years are expected to participate in the practice exercises only. The groups are structured, however, to help children remain attentive by asking relevant questions and actively engaging them in the process.

3. High Noise/Activity Levels Within Groups

The current multiple-family group incorporates family members at differing developmental levels. MFTGs are facilitated based upon the assumption that the group will manage its own activity level as parents are expected to address the behavior of their children at home. Therefore, parents have direct opportunities to help children manage their volume and behavior level during the group.

4. Content Around Race/Poverty/Community Must Be Incorporated

Each of the group members must parent within a context that is influenced by racism, poverty, and community violence. Not only do these issues need to be understood by the group facilitators, they need to be addressed as serious barriers to effective, nurturant parenting. Portions of the group are often focused on the impact of the environment on parents and children. As group facilitators grow more aware of the importance of these issues, they will provide more opportunities for their discussion, as demonstrated in the following:

> During the initial meeting, facilitated by a white worker, an African-American single mother began to discuss her own experience as a grade school student. She described herself as being an unmotivated student who left school after her junior year. She focused on a teacher who she described as "possibly prejudiced." She cited an example of the teacher ignoring minority students, but immediately followed this by questioning whether her perceptions were accurate. The worker responded by clearly identifying school systems as reflecting racism that exists within the larger society. In fact, the worker cited past examples from other families where the children had not been treated fairly because of the color of their skin. The mother in the group expressed agreement with the worker's comments and began to discuss some of her own concerns about her son's interaction with a principal and her fears about approaching the school on his behalf.

The incorporation of an understanding of how a parent's context influences the ability to parent is critical to developing a therapeutic multiple-family group for inner-city families.

CONCLUSION

The use of MFTGs has shown promise in motivating families to remain actively involved in treatment. Families identify increased feelings of support and a decreased sense of isolation through their participation with other families. In addition, parents frequently express their appreciation for having the opportunity to listen to their children and receive feedback from families facing the same issues and concerns.

The facilitation of multiple-family groups is not without its obstacles, as outlined above. From a clinical perspective, the benefits outweigh these challenges. Future attention of practitioners need now to turn toward more rigorously evaluating the usefulness of MFTGs in relation to other, more established treatment modalities. One of the greatest obstacles to such evaluation is differentiating the impact of participation in the multiple-family group when a family is also involved in other services at an agency. Furthermore, applying the conceptual framework that change occurs within the multiple-family group and individual family units at multiple levels presents significant barriers to empirically defining the process of change.

Multiple-family groups show promise in assisting families in addressing parenting concerns. Regular attendance throughout these groups, along with consistently positive evaluations by other parents, have given support for the need to refine this treatment modality further.

BIBLIOGRAPHY

Acosta, F.X. (1980). Self-Described Reasons for Premature Termination of Psychotherapy by Mexican American, Black American and Anglo-American Patients. *Psychological Reports*, 47: 435-443.

Anderson, C.M. (1986). A Psychoeducational Program for Families of Patients with Schizophrenia. *Family Therapy in Schizophrenia*, New York: Guilford Press.

Anton, R., Hogan Z., Jalali, B., Riodan, C., and Kleber, H. (1981). Multiple Family Therapy and Naltrexone in the Treatment of Opiate Dependence. *Drug and Alcohol Dependence*, 8: 157-168.

Aponte, H.J., Zarski, J., Bixenstene, C., and Cibik, P. (1991). Home/Community-Based Services: A Two-Tier Approach. *American Journal of Orthopsychiatry*, 61(3): 403-408.

Brandenburg, N.A., Friedman, R.M., and Silver, S.E. (1987). The Epidemiology of Childhood Psychiatric Disorders: Prevalence Findings from Recent Studies. *Journal of the American Academy of Child and Adolescent Psychiatry*, 29: 76-83.

Bruenlin, D., Schwartz, R., and Karrer, B. (1993). *Metaframework*. California: Jossey-Bass, Inc.

Boyd-Franklin, N. (1993). Black Families. In Walsh, Froma (Ed.), *Normal Family Process*. New York: Guilford Press.

Cassano, D.R. (1989a). Multi-Family Group Therapy in Social Work Practice-Part I. *Social Work with Groups,* 12(1), 3-14. Binghamton, NY: The Haworth Press, Inc.

Cassano, D.R. (1989b). The Multi-Family Therapy Group: Research on Patterns of Interaction-Part II. *Social Work with Groups,* 12(1), 15-39. Binghamton, NY: The Haworth Press, Inc.

Cheung, F.K. and Snowden, L.R. (1989). Utilization of Inpatient Services by Members of Ethnic Minority Groups. Paper presented at Oklahoma Mental Health Research Institute Professional Symposium, Tulsa, OK.

Curry, A.E. (1965). Management of Multiple Family Groups. *International Journal of Group Psychotherapy,* 15: 90-96.

Falloon, I.R.H., Liberman, R., Lellie, I., and Vaughn, I. (1981). Family Therapy of Schizophrenia with High Risk of Relapse. *Family Process,* 20: 211-223.

Falloon, I., and Liberman, R. (1983). Behavioral Family Intervention in the Management of Chronic Schizophrenia in W.R. McFarlane (Ed.), *Family Therapy in Schizophrenia.*

Flaskerud, J.H. (1986). The Effects of Culture-Compatible Intervention on the Utilization of Mental Health Services by Minority Clients. *Community Mental Health Journal,* 22(2): 127-140.

Foley, V.D. (1982). Multiple Family Therapy with Urban Blacks. In L.A. Wolberg and M.L. Aronson (Eds.). *Group and Family Therapy.* New York: Brunner/Mazel.

Gary, L.E. (1982). Attitude Toward Human Service Organizations: Perspectives from an Urban Black Community. *Journal Of Applied Behavioral Sciences,* 21: 445-458.

Gould, E. and Glick, I.D. (1977). The Effects of Family Presence and Brief Family Intervention on Global Outcome for Hospitalized Schizophrenic Patients. *Family Process,* 16: 503-510.

Gould, E. and Degroot, D. (1981). Inter and Intrafamily Interaction in Multifamily Group Therapy. *American Journal of Family Therapy,* 9: 65-74.

Guerra, N., Huessman, R., Tolan, P., Van Acker, R., and Eror, L. (1990). *Metropolitan Area Child Study Grant Proposal.* National Institute of Mental Health.

Hardcastle, D.R. (1977). A Multiple Family Counseling Program: Procedures and Results. *Family Process,* 16: 67-74.

Kadis, L.B. and McClendon, R.A. (1981). Redecision Family Therapy: Its use with Intensive Multiple Family Groups. *The American Journal of Family Therapy,* 9(2): 75-83.

Kazdin, A. (1993). Premature Termination from Treatment Among Children Referred for antisocial Behavior. *Journal of Clinical Child Psychology,* 31(8): 415-425.

Keefe, S.E., Padilla, A.M., and Carlos, M.L. (1979). The Mexican-American Extended Family as an Emotional Support System. *Human Organization,* 38: 144-152.

Laqueur, H.P. (1976). Multiple Family Therapy. In Guerin, P.J. (Ed), *Family Therapy Theory and Practice.* New York: Gardner. 405-416.

Laqueur, H.P. (1980). The Theory and Practice of Multiple Family Therapy. *Group and Family Therapy*, 5, 15-23.

Leichter, E. and Schulman, G.L. (1972). Interplay of Group and Family Treatment, Techniques in Multi-Family Group Therapy. *International Journal of Group Psychotherapy*, 22: 167-176.

Leichter, E. and Schulman, G.L. (1981). Multi-Family Group Therapy: A Multidimensional Approach. *Family Process*, 13: 1-13.

Leichter, E. and Schulman, G.L. (1986). Emerging Phenomena in Multi-Family Group Treatment. *International Journal of Group Psychotherapy*, 18: 59-69.

Leichter, E. and Schulman, G.L. (1986). Emerging Phenomena in Multi-Family Group Treatment. *International Journal of Group Psychotherapy*, 18: 59-69.

Libo, S.S., Palmer, C. and Archibald, D. (1971). Family Group Therapy for Children with Self-Induced Seizures. *American Journal of Orthopsychiatry*, 41(3): 506-509.

Lin, T. (1983). Psychiatry and Chinese Culture. *Western Journal of Medicine*, 139: 868-874.

Muecke, M.A. (1983). In Search of Healers–Southeast Asia Refugees in the American Health Care System. *Western Journal of Medicine*, 139: 835-840.

O'Shea, M. and Phelps, R. (1985). Multiple Family Therapy: Current Status and Critical Appraisal. *Family Process*, 24: 555-582.

Patterson, G. and Forgatch, M. (1987). *Parents and Adolescents Living Together*. Eugene, OR: Castalia Publishing Company.

Paul, N.L., Brool, J. and Paul, B. (1980). Outpatient Multiple Family Group Therapy–Why Not? In L.R. Walberg and M.L. Aronson (Eds.), *Group and Family Therapy*. New York: Brunner/Mazel.

Reiss, D. and Costell, R. (1977). The Multiple Family Group as a Small Society: Family Regulation of Interaction with Nonmembers. *American Journal of Psychiatry*, 134: 21-24.

Rhodes, R.M. and Zelman, A.B. (1986). An On Going Multi-Family Group in a Women's Shelter. *American Journal of Orthopsychiatry*, 56 (1): 120-130.

Sue, S. (1977). Community Mental Health Services to Minority Groups. *American Psychologist*, 32: 616-624.

Strelnick, A. (1978). Multiple Family Group Therapy: A Review of the Literature. *Family Process*, 307-325.

Szymanski, L.S. and Kiernan, W. (1983). Multiple Family Group Therapy with Developmentally Disabled Adolescents and Young Adults. *International Journal of Group Psychotherapy*, 33 (4): 521-534.

Tolan, P. and Gorman-Smith, D. (1991). *Parenting Questionnaire*. Chicago, IL: University of Illinois at Chicago.

Tolan, P. and Gorman-Smith, D. (1991). *Stress Questionnaire*. Chicago, IL: University of Illinois at Chicago.

Tolan, P., Florsheim, P., McKay, M., and Kohner, K. (1993). Metropolitan *Area Child Study Family Intervention Manual*. Chicago, IL: University of Illinois.

Tuma, J.M. (1989). Mental Health Services for Children. *American Psychologist*, 46: 188-189.

Chapter 8

Horizontes: Using Social Work with Groups in the Classroom to Serve the Needs of Latino College Students

Flavio Francisco Marsiglia

STATEMENT OF THE PROBLEM

Hispanic Americans are the fastest growing ethnic minority and speakers of the second most prevalent language in this country. According to the 1990 U.S. Census, 139,696 of the 22 million Hispanics counted in the United States were residing in Ohio. The state's Latino population was younger than any other group–37.6 percent were under 18 years old. Nearly 74 percent of Ohio Latinos (97,600) were concentrated in the 21 northern counties of the state. Cuyahoga County had the largest concentration of Hispanics (31,447) with Puerto Ricans as the largest Latino subgroup. Between 1980 and 1990 the Latino population of the city of Cleveland alone experienced an impressive 30.5 percent growth, while the city's white population decreased by 18.5 percent and the African-American population decreased by 6.3 percent.

Nationally, in 1990, Hispanic Americans were 9 percent of the U.S. population while representing only 5.6 percent of higher education enrollment.[1] This situation is showing some improvement. Since 1987, the number of Latinos receiving an associate degree has risen by 16 percent nationwide. Between 1980 and 1990 the number of Latinos enrolled in Ohio's two-year, post-secondary institutions grew by 61.8 percent (from 1,069 students in 1980 to 1,773 students in 1990), representing 1.1 percent of the total Ohio enrollment for two-year institutions.[2] Despite these improvements, Ohio Latinos remain underrepresented at the state's two-year institutions.

Of particular concern is the very low rate of degree completion achieved by Latinos. In point of fact, Hispanic-American students are dropping out of school at alarming rates. Thirty-five percent of all 16- to 24-year-old Latinos in the United States were classified as high-school dropouts in 1991.[3] They are among the non-native English-speaking students who, generally, have historically been dropping out of school at rates three to four times higher than native English speakers (Kyle, 1984).

Latino students attending the Cleveland City School District follow national Latino dropout trends. A study using the cohort method to calculate the district's dropout rate (Cataldo, 1990) reported that 34.5 percent of all Latinos (and 26.1 percent of all African-Americans) enrolled in the ninth grade in 1984 dropped out before graduation. Socioeconomic barriers must also be considered. Nationally, 37.7 percent of Hispanic children live in poverty, while in the city of Cleveland the percentage rises to 47.4 percent. Many of these children may be at risk of school failure. Without adequate intervention and support, many will not be prepared for college. Reported high dropout rates and low socioeconomic status continue to drastically decimate the pool of candidates for post-secondary education in the city of Cleveland and in the county of Cuyahoga.

More than 500 Latino students were enrolled in Cuyahoga Community College in 1992. Historically, a very small percentage of all the Latino students enrolled graduate in two years, transfer to other post-secondary institutions, or remain enrolled at Cuyahoga Community College. It is against this background that the Horizontes Project was conceived.

REVIEW OF THE LITERATURE

Culture has been broadly used to explain the poor performance of Hispanics in school as well as their low visibility in other institutions. According to the prevailing stereotype, Hispanics are perceived to be noncompetitive, non future-oriented, and family-centered. These attributes are commonly seen as all but ensuring poor performance in school (Bean and Tienda, 1987). While the reality of cultural differences cannot be denied, a more perceptive interpretation of the impact these factors have in the academic life of Hispanic students is needed. Special attention must be given to the cultural conflict Hispanic students experience as they are forced to become bicultural with respect to learning processes, communication styles, and human relations in general.

Schools rarely accommodate this duality. As agents of socialization, specifically Americanization, schools and colleges have been the explicit site for cultural homogenization and dilution of ethnic identity. Cultural denigration, when it occurs and is internalized by Hispanic students, translates into low self-esteem and further contributes to low achievement (Bean and Tienda, 1987). Moreover, the Latino student body is a very heterogenous group. Simplistic generalizations must be avoided. In Cleveland's case, Puerto Rican students constitute a distinct population deserving of special attention.

First under Spanish and later under the American rule, Puerto Rico has never been an independent nation. Bird (1982) has illustrated how individual self-definition, self-esteem, and ethnic identity have been negatively affected by the colonial experience. In addition, Puerto Ricans are the first group to come to the mainland in large numbers and from a different cultural background who are nevertheless already citizens of the United States. Since their first days on the mainland, Puerto Ricans have tended to maintain closer than usual contact with their island communities of origin. They have accomplished this through a complex pattern of migration and reverse migration. The contact flow between the island and the mainland and the reverse migration yield a uniquely Puerto Rican transculturation, involving both adaptive and re-adaptive processes (Comas-Díaz, 1987).

This circular migration means that the island population and mainland community are two parts of one whole, a situation that distinguishes Puerto Ricans from other Hispanic-American subgroups and other minority groups. An effect of this circular migration is that elements of both cultures thrive in both places, a feat that requires dual functional abilities. Students in this subculture must be able to switch language and school systems and must cope with competing value systems. Constant transition from one culture to another has produced a condition of marginality that is stressful and often conducive to mental breakdown (Badillo-Ghali, 1977). On the other hand, this persistence of ethnic distinctiveness, despite massive pressure to conform to the homogeneous consumer culture, has been interpreted by some authors as a form of protest (specifically, Nelson and Tienda, 1985).

The specialized literature has identified several cultural descriptors as unique to the Puerto Rican case. Of these, the Puerto Rican language/culture continuum has received the most attention. Flores, Attinasi, and Pedraza Jr. (1981), in his East Harlem study explained the concept of a Puerto Rican language spectrum as characterized by a bilingual range with a colonial dialect at each of the two poles. The Puerto-Rican Spanish pole, with its admixture of indigenous, African, and peasant qualities, is stigmatized to this day as a corruption of the pure mother tongue and other, supposedly more faithful, Latin American variants. The other pole represents the acquired language, a blend of the urban varieties of American English most immediately accessible to Puerto Ricans. This may also be seen by the majority society as a downgraded dialect, distinct from, but sharing much with, "black English." In cities with large African-American communities, Latino students tend to incorporate a good deal of the African-American urban dialect and other cultural identifiers seen by such students as "American" (Marsiglia, 1991).

Most Puerto Ricans in mainland United States are not located at either of these two poles, but fall somewhere between them. The resulting phenomenon is the interpenetrating usage of both languages–derogatorily called "Spanglish"–in a wide range of circumstances. It is especially useful for in-group communication. The East Harlem study concluded that a highly adaptive phenomenon referred to as code-switching represents neither the lack of language nor structural convergence. Rather, it often signals an expansion of communicative and expressive potential. The presence of "loan" words was identified as the most visible aspect of language contact, and it was explained as part of every kind of contact between cultures. Harding and Riley (1986) explained code-switching as a phenomenon that is limited to bilingual situations, where bilinguals talk to other bilinguals and where they can call upon the full communicative resources of both languages.

Traditional ESL Programs

English as a Second Language (ESL) teaching in the United States has traditionally been based on the described "assimilationist" model. That is to say, the acquisition of English is the key to accessing the benefits of mainstream American society (McKay, 1988). Students are, therefore, to be assimilated into the majority culture as rapidly and as completely as possible. ESL is often taught with no support from the first language and with no regard for the student's native culture. This has been particularly true at the college level, where the aim has usually been to move the students into an academic program in English as soon as possible. Because college students often come from a number of linguistic and cultural backgrounds, it is considered expedient to mix them together in a single class where English is the "working language." Some teachers still forbid the use of native languages in such classes. The assimilationist model has been the basis for the ESL curriculum at Cuyahoga Community College since such classes were first offered in the late 1960s.

Flaws in the model only became apparent as the student population of the college began to change over the years as more and more minority students (e.g., Hispanic and Asian) enrolled in ESL programs. The assimilationist model claims that the process of learning English is the same for all students. It denies historical inequalities that exist among cultural groups. There is no regard for differences in learning styles, socioeconomic background, or minority status. The method is the same for all. Cambodians, Puerto Ricans, Ukrainians, and Saudi Arabians are all expected to learn in exactly the same way and even at the same speed. According to N. Clair (1994),

> believing that English is the sole indicator that separates language minority students' ability to successfully enter the American mainstream ignores the social and political reality within which language-minority students exist. It denies the existence of racism and social inequalities that have been historic realities for many immigrant (and migrant) groups. (p. 9)

Studies in bilingualism have clearly shown that first-language development supports second-language development and that knowledge is transferrable between languages (Ovando and Collier, 1985). It has become evident that bilingualism is both desirable and useful to the student and to society. The "pluralistic" notion of language-learning not only permits the use of the first language, but encourages it as a means to motivate the student. Content is especially important in learning a second language. If the learner perceives the content of a lesson to be relevant, learner motivation will be high (Brinton, Snow, and Wesche 1989). In addition, language must be used for authentic purposes if it is to be learned. Repetitive exercises with little relevance to the students' lives are of little value. From these principles arise the notion of tapping into the students' native culture and areas of natural interest and using cultural content in order to motivate them to learn English.

THEORETICAL APPROXIMATION TO THE PROBLEM

American postsecondary educators (product of a monolingual educational system) face the challenge of recognizing bilingual Puerto Rican/Latino students as linguistically competent students. Language competence, in a Chomskian sense, means that all individuals are biologically endowed with the faculty of language (Chomsky, 1968). The "surface structure" of the students' speech may be labeled at times as Puerto-Rican Spanish, black English, "Spanglish," or standard English. However, the "deep structure" of their speech reflects the substantive and formal universality of language. Integrating multiculturalism and valuing bilingualism in the classroom will assist educators to work with the two structures of the students' speech and become more effective in reaching out to the Latino student.

Postsecondary institutions have a very important role to play as agents of assimilation of minority students into the mainstream society and its benefits. Assimilation, however, is understood here as a dynamic process rooted in the student's unique historical processes and cultures (Vygostky, 1979). Services and programs designed to meet the needs of Puerto-Rican/Latino students should provide a space where students are able to combine their spontaneous concepts–those based on cultural and social practices–with those introduced by teachers in the instructional setting (Freire, 1970). Students who find their culture and learning styles reflected in both the substance and the organization of the instructional program are more likely to be motivated and to benefit from their learning experience (Kuykendall, 1992).

In summary, there is a need to (1) recognize the richness of students' culture, and (2) direct existing "cultural/linguistic tools" toward the full achievement of students' potential. To address these needs, faculty and other staff have to be trained or retrained to become more sensitive to the needs and assets brought to the classroom by Latino students. The college has to provide a "safe"learning environment, with support services in place that will make Latino students feel welcome and a part of the college community.

PROJECT HORIZONTES

Background

In Spring 1992, under the auspices of the Cuyahoga Community College's Hispanic Council, a series of site visits were made to colleges where Latino programs were in place or where there were significant Latino enrollments. The purpose of these visits was to become familiar with existing models.

During the summer of 1992, a group social worker was hired as a consultant to work with a group of Cuyahoga Community College (CCC) ESL teachers. Some of the teachers had expressed concern about the college's lack of effectiveness in reaching the Latino students, other teachers became part of the group due to their administrative responsibilities over curriculum. The team agreed to meet with the social worker/consultant in order to determine the need and design a pilot project that would help them to better serve the needs of Latino students attending CCC's metro campus.

The team operated as a focus group and later as the project design team. Although the faculty group operated as a "task group," it quickly developed into a growth and support type of group. During the initial sessions the topics of discussion were centered around

Puerto Rican/Latino cultures, students' learning styles, and the status of Puerto Rican/Latino students attending the college. Instructors started to analyze their own perceptions and biases in a non-hierarchical way. As the group process developed, the intensity and depth of the discussions increased. Members not only became more aware of the problem, they started to question each other's attitudes and behaviors toward the Latino students. The team came to the following conclusion:

> Puerto Rican/Latino students enrolled in Cuyahoga Community College have disproportionately low retention and academic success rates. Their diverse cultural and linguistic backgrounds have not been systematically recognized and/or integrated in the past as resources for their academic success. A pervasive lack of recognition of their cultural distinctiveness has had a negative influence on their attitudes toward college education. These students often perceive the College as an uncaring environment where they are not welcome.

The team recommended that a culturally grounded ESL pilot program be designed and implemented in response to the identified needs.

Project Description

Project Horizontes (horizons) was designed as a culturally based ESL program to serve the unique needs of the Puerto Rican/Latino students enrolled at the metro campus of Cuyahoga Community College. Horizontes was intended to provide Latino students enrolled in ESL courses with a culturally relevant support system that would enable them to have an academically challenging and rewarding college entry experience. A description of the project is as follows:

Project Purpose: To increase the retention rate of Puerto Rican/ Latino students enrolled in Cuyahoga Community College-metro campus.

Desired Outcomes: 1. At least 70 percent of the students enrolled will successfully complete the program and will enroll in the following quarter.
2. At least 80 percent of the students will have a 90 percent or higher attendance rate.

Approach: Collaborative learning, team teaching, small class size, and psycho-social support–academically challenging, culturally grounded, holistic, and bilingual.

Project Design

Students enrolled in Horizontes are exposed to a variety of activities. In terms of course-work, a bilingual approach is being taken in two of the three courses, and all three courses are bicultural in content. Those courses are described here:

1. In the all-Latino ESL 112 writing course, the instructor is bilingual, and Spanish is used to reinforce concepts learned in English.
2. The core group of Latino students is divided in two subgroups, and they are placed with other ESL students in two ESL 111 classes taught by project team members. This intermediate ESL grammar course is taught in English with some limited reinforcement in Spanish.
3. An all-Latino SP 243 course (4 hours per week) is taught in Spanish and uses social work with group modality. Latino cultural awareness is emphasized, using short stories in Spanish (see Appendix A for List of Readings). Students receive foreign language credits upon completion, which can be transferred to a four-year college.

The Latino culture course (SP 243) focuses exclusively on Latino studies, alongside the other two ESL courses. Participants in the program are part of the whole language and culture continuum: Spanish-Latino culture to English-American culture. The Latino culture instructor introduces the topic of the week (e.g., machismo, fatalism, the Latino family), and the other two instructors use those concepts and materials introduced in the Latino culture course in their ESL classes. Thus, the content of the ESL classes becomes culturally relevant for the student. Topics are illustrated with short stories written by young Latin-American writers (mostly female and Puerto Rican).

Other Activities

Support Groups/Mentorship

A faculty member identifies and trains Horizontes' graduates as peer facilitators to lead groups formed by new project participants. The groups meet every other week. Small groups use English, Spanish, or both languages according to need. The faculty member supports the peer facilitators and acts as a supervisor. The peer facilitators receive a stipend for their work.

Social Activities, Lectures, and Luncheon Forums

At least one of these activities is presented each month. All students are invited to participate. In some instances, guest speakers are invited. Themes are related to ethnic identity, the college experience, or special culturally relevant celebrations.

Biweekly Faculty Meetings

These meetings are used to (a) monitor and assess the programmatic aspects of the project, (b) coordinate lesson plans under common themes, and (c) assess the progress of individual students.

SOCIAL WORK WITH GROUPS IN THE CLASSROOM

The Latino culture class is in fact an educational/growth group (as defined by Toseland and Rivas, 1995). Students are informed about the modality used in this course during orientation and registration. If they decide to enroll in the Horizontes Project, they need to take the Latino culture class. They have the option to register in the regular ESL courses.

The course is structured in such a way that the different stages of group development can be followed. During the beginning phase, rules such as confidentiality are discussed and goals are agreed upon. The students develop a contract and assess it throughout the working phase. At the end of the quarter, they write a paper outlining what they learned and their short- and long-range goals. This "final paper" aims to assist the group members to arrive at a planned termination phase.

During the working stage, a topic is discussed in each session. Students come prepared to discuss a particular topic related to Latino culture. The sessions are organized as follows:

A. Warm-Up/Sharing Period (20 minutes)

Students share with each other events and experiences they had during the week.

B. Presentation of the Topic by the Teacher/Facilitator (30 minutes)

For example, the topic of the week may be "fatalism." The instructor provides the content from a culturally grounded perspective and using a postmodern feminist approach (Sands and Nuccio, 1992). The presentation aims to regain ownership of the cultural descriptor providing a focus for discussion. The presentation is interactive in nature and introduces "words" and "meaning." José, one of the participants, commented,

> Mucho le agradezco al profesor por darnos vocabulario que nunca habíamos oído en nuestras vidas. (Many thanks to the instructor for giving us a vocabulary that we've never heard before in our lives.)

Learning and incorporating this vocabulary provides the participants with a sense of ownership and control over their lives. They are not diagnosing, they are interpreting. Students quickly incorporate the terminology and use it with each other. Stephanie expressed her ideas about fatalism, as follows:

> Del cuento, aprendí que uno no debe ser fatalista. No importa cual sea el problema, sea grande o pequeño, cada uno de nosotros tenemos oportunidades de buscar una solución. (From the short story, I learned that one can't be a fatalist. It doesn't matter what type of a problem we may face, it could be

big or little, each one of us has opportunities to look for a solution.)

As part of the group process, members start to identify and name behaviors. They begin to "discover" names for resources and barriers present in their culture.

C. One of the Students Presents the Short Story Assigned for That Session (20 minutes)

The readings are the program activities. The Latino culture is a literary culture; Puerto Rican culture is not an exception. Most of the stories used are written by young female Puerto Rican writers, and the authors can be described as part of the "magic realism" movement. The presenter is viewed by the group as a resource, he or she is expected to facilitate the group's search for meaning, understanding, and interpretation of the short story's symbology.

The short stories provide a culturally grounded context in which to discuss important issues. Although there is a clear feminist approach in the members' analysis of certain topics, it is not an Anglo middle-class approach. Luz commented after presenting a short story to the group:

> Esta historia nos enseña valores; por ejemplo, que las mujeres se hagan respetar por los hombres para que ellos no piensen que pueden jugar con las mujeres. Tenemos que empezar a tener respeto por una misma para que los hombres nos respeten y nos valoren; es decir, darnos el lugar o el puesto que nos corresponde. (The story teaches us values; for example, that women need to make men respect them, so that they stop thinking that they can mess with women. We need to start having respect for ourselves so that they will start to respect and value us; in other words, give us the place or position we deserve.)

The "voice" of the writer and her characters become a source of inspiration and often serve as a role model.

D. Integration/Personalization/Universalization (45 minutes)

Students learn how to connect the story with the topic of the week. They identify with a character or characters of the short story.

The topic takes on a human dimension. Students find commonalities with those characters and their own lives. They also find commonalities among themselves and discover the "universality" of the issues being discussed. In her final paper María wrote,

> As Hispanic students, we often underestimate ourselves and feel intimidated by others. We must be realistic and accept that we will overcome the language barrier someday.

In one of the group sessions Aracelis added,

> En la universidad, no por el color de mi piel, sino porque al no saber inglés me siento inferior a los demas y no me siento entre los míos. Pero en el grupo, me siento entre los míos, porque todos conocemos la cultura, sabemos el idioma . . . (In the college, not because of the color of my skin but because I don't understand English, I feel inferior to other people and don't feel among my people. But in the group, I feel like I am among my own, we all know the the culture, language . . .)

By participating in the group, the students internalize that they are not alone or "strange." They develop alternatives and start to model new behaviors in the safety of the group. Mariccelli's comment illustrates this concept:

> I have learned in group that we have to try harder sometimes because we are Hispanic. We need to be together, like a family. I would like to see us as one, staying together and succeeding.

As the process of mutual aid begins, a sense of accountability toward the group starts to emerge. Culture is celebrated and begins to be used as a resource to improve the students' quality of life here and now. In the last session of her group, Carmen said,

> Como mujer y mujer hispana puedo lograr muchos cambios y lograr una vida mejor, no solo para mí sino tambien para mi comunidad. Si yo soy feliz, todas las personas a mi alrededor podrán compartir esta felicidad." (As a woman, a Hispanic woman, I can make many changes and attain a better life, not

only for me but also for my community. If I am happy, everyone around me can share in that happiness.)

The group work modality in the Latino culture component provides a space in which to try new behaviors of participation, expression, and decision-making. Students experience the democratic process in the group and develop skills that they can use in other environments. Katherine expressed this process in her own terms:

Como estudiante Latina, siento aún una mayor responsibilidad de expresar y defender mis ideales. Pues, al ser minoría siento que debo hacerme escuchar, solo así podré defender, mantener, y poner mi raza, mi cultura, y mis ideales en alto. (As a Latina student, I feel an even greater responsibility to express and defend my ideals. Because I'm considered minority, I feel like I have to make myself listen because only then will I be able to defend, maintain, and put my race, my culture, and my ideals in the forefront.)

Leadership skills developed or reinforced in the group are used by the students serving as peer facilitators, running for office in college organizations, and getting involved in community organizations. In group, they feel as the adults they are. In their language they are able to express important ideas. Those ideas are then transferred and translated into the English classes, providing meaningful content to the otherwise tedious and child-like courses.

The next section will provide some outcome data gathered and analyzed during the pilot phase of the project.

ASSESSMENT OF PILOT PHASE

This section reports only on the project's pilot phase during the 1992 fall quarter and the 1993 winter quarter. During that period, a total of 26 Latino students successfully completed the program. All project-desired outcomes were attained.

Desired Outcome 1: At least 70 percent of the students enrolled will successfully complete the program and will be enrolled in the following quarter.

Desired Outcome 1 was attained. High percentages of participants completed the program and enrolled in the following quarter/s. (See Tables 8.1 and 8.2.)

As Table 8.1 illustrates, the project's overall 89 percent retention rate surpassed the desired outcome by 19 percentage points. Table 8.2 illustrates the college retention rate of project participants.

TABLE 8.1. Quarter Completion Rate

	Fall 1992	Winter 1993	Overall
Started	19	10	29
Dropped	1	2	3
Difference	18	8	26
Retention Rate	(94%)	(80%)	**(89%)**

TABLE 8.2. College Retention Rate

	Fall 1992	Winter 1993	Spring 1993
1st Cohort	19 (100%)	16 (84%)	12 (63%)
2nd Cohort		10 (100%)	8 (80%)

The high mobility rate that characterized Puerto Rican students lowered the "real" survival rate of the first cohort. Notwithstanding, both student cohorts achieved a college survival rate well beyond the level established by the desired outcome.

Desired Outcome 2: At least 80 percent of the students will have a 90 percent or higher attendance rate. This desired outcome was attained by project participants as a whole, but it was not attained by the winter quarter cohort. Table 8.3 illustrates the differences found between the fall and winter cohorts.

The severity of the weather was identified by faculty members as a determining factor explaining the lower average attendance rate attained by winter cohort participants. The desired outcome was attained by project participants when both cohorts' attendance rates were combined.

The primary purpose of this program was to improve retention of Latino college students. A high 89 percent overall quarter completion rate was attained during the pilot, as compared with the goal set of a 70 percent quarter completion rate. College persistence at the metro cam-

TABLE 8.3. Attendance Rate (N = 26)

	Total N	N with 90% Attendance	Percent (%)
Fall 1992	18	16	88.8
Winter 1993	8	5	62.5
Overall	26	21	**80.7**
Attendance Rate	(94%)	(80%)	**(89%)**

pus of Cuyahoga Community College, as measured by the rate of re-enrollment, was in the 80 percent range after one quarter and in the 60 percent range after two quarters, as compared with faculty estimates of approximately 20 percent after two quarters prior to the Horizontes program. This result was achieved in spite of the fact that it was not possible to follow up with non-reregistering students to find out how many re-enrolled at another branch of CCC, other mainland U.S. institutions, or–as is known to be true in at least one case–at Puerto Rican institutions of higher education, all of which could fairly be defined as evidence of college persistence.

Additional Findings

Additional indicators were analyzed to complement the data gathered while assessing the project's desired outcomes. These additional indicators included participants' grades, attitudes, and language skills.

Grades

Table 8.4 presents the average grade point of both participating cohorts of students.

As Table 8.4 illustrates, overall, grade point averages fluctuated within the C range (2 to 2.7 points). In both cohorts, over 50 percent of the students had final grades ranging from C to A.

Language Skills

The project incorporated a new multidimensional curriculum, however, the ultimate purpose of ESL courses continued to be to assist students to advance in their English language development. Table 8.5 presents the results of pre- and post-test administered to a cohort of participants.

A difference of 3.5 points can be interpreted as an important gain in terms of language skills. Besides these gains, there was considerable evidence to indicate that significant learning took place. This evidence includes the following:

- Self-reports by students that they learned a lot in the way of grammar, writing, vocabulary, and comprehension

- One faculty report stating "These students definitely worked harder in general than most other Hispanic students I have taught at Cuyahoga Community College" and several reports that students supported each other in mastering course content both in and out of class to an unusual degree
- Pre- Post-English-Test results (an objective measure of achievement) showing a 33 percent improvement
- Grades for the two courses that were within the C to A range targeted for the project

Attitude

A locally constructed scale was used to assess changes in the students' attitudes toward college. (See Appendix B for a copy of

TABLE 8.4. Grade-Point Average (N = 26)

	ESL 111	ESL 112	Overall
First Cohort	2.3	2.6	2.5
Second Cohort	1.7	3.2	2.0
Overall	2.1	2.7	**2.4**

TABLE 8.5. Language Closed-Test Average Scores (N = 18)

	Pretest	Posttest	Difference
Average Scores	10.5	14.0	**3.5**

the instrument.) Students were asked to rate a set of statements written in English and Spanish using a Likert scale (1 = strongly disagree to 5 = strongly agree). Questionnaires were administered to the two cohorts during the first week and last week of each quarter (pre- and post-tests). Items rated in reverse were adjusted for the analysis. Table 8.6 presents the students' average scores for fall and winter quarters and an overall cumulative set of average scores.

Table 8.6 illustrates that there were almost no differences between the pre- and post-test cumulative scores. The assumption is that Latino students enrolled in the program were motivated and wanted to succeed, as reflected by a 3.5 cumulative average score. It can be surmised that project participation assisted Latino students in maintaining a moderately positive initial attitude toward college.

An item analysis identified items d, f, h, and i as the items presenting the greater score differences.

Item f: "I feel uncomfortable speaking English."
           A difference of −.8 can be interpreted as a reflection of the confidence students gained in their ability to communicate in English within a "safe" environment.
Item h: "I get nervous when participating in class."
           The change in attitude mentioned for item f may also be reflected in the −.4 difference registered for this item.
Item i: "I feel good when I am with other Hispanics."
           A difference of +.5 can be interpreted as a benefit gained from the support received from fellow Latinos. Students developed a true support system among themselves that appeared to have prevented the development of a sense of isolation experienced by other Latino students not enrolled in the project.
Item d: "Personal problems do not let me advance."
           A difference of +.5 may reflect the respondents' greater awareness about the relationship between their personal lives and their education.

The Latino culture component of the project dealt with this relationship from a culturally specific perspective. This awareness level was followed up with specific efforts toward attitude and behavior

TABLE 8.6. Attitudinal Survey Average Scores (N=26)

	Pretest	Posttest	Difference
First Cohort	3.6	3.7	.1
Second Cohort	3.4	3.4	---
Overall	3.5	3.6	.1

modification. These efforts were intended to help students gain a greater sense of control over their own lives.

Attitude, as measured by the pre- post-test attitude surveys, remained constant and reasonably positive throughout the program. This was interpreted as significant since the previously high dropout rate was accompanied by a good deal of discouragement on the part of many Hispanic students. According to faculty reports, students ended up feeling like they "didn't fit in." Another indication of the attitude change of participants was the high seriousness of purpose reflected in the many comments on feedback sheets requesting more grammar, more writing, more vocabulary, and more emphasis on English.

The impact of the project during the pilot phase was clearly positive. Several questions remain about factors contributing to the success of the pilot and adjustments that could further enhance its effectiveness in the future. Several of these are discussed below.

The most important theoretical assumption underlying the program was that a strong commitment to recognizing, respecting, and enhancing bilingualism would accelerate and reinforce "positive assimilation." This was translated into the design of the program primarily through the bilingual content and the bilingual communication/interaction patterns established in ESL 112, and through bilingual communication in the support groups. Latinos were not punished for or discouraged from speaking Spanish. The level of comfort established is reflected by the fact that some students filled out the course evaluation forms partly in English and partly in Spanish.

It is also clear that the strong support system for Hispanic students developed in the program contributed substantially to improved retention and academic performance. It can be surmised that the social work with group modality strengthened and supported a natural culturally grounded tendency toward group solidarity. Without the program, entry-level students would have not had the opportunity to be together and "connect" with each other. It is difficult to ascertain the relative importance of respective design elements in the absence of controls. (It appears a likely, although as yet untested, hypothesis that the combination of factors employed produced a better result than any one factor or element might have generated alone.)

At a deeper level, it is possible to question just how fully the concept of "bilingualism as an expansion of expressive capabilities" has been implemented into the design of the Horizontes program. While student use of Spanish was corrected in papers and during oral presentations and interaction, would a simultaneous course in the Spanish language (as contrasted with Latino culture), have represented a more forceful commitment to enhanced bilingualism? A stronger commitment to enhancing Spanish language fluency would not only further enhance self-image, but also further develop competence in the "language of grammar" and the "language of language learning," mentioned by faculty as needing further attention. Involving Latino students as tutors in such classes would also be a possibility.

The importance of this bilingualism to our society, and not just to the individuals in question, may be illustrated if we consider the potential value added to the international business capabilities of the United States if bilingualism is truly enhanced rather than viewed as a passing phase and then implicitly extinguished through neglect. For example, most Russian immigrants no longer speak Russian. However, a number of families remaining active in the Russian Orthodox Church kept language fluency alive. These people, today, are playing leadership roles in establishing business ties with the new republics of the former Soviet Union.

Generally speaking, there appeared to be two responses to the design of the program, depending on the amount of time students had been living in mainland United States prior to enrollment. Those new to the mainland tended to appreciate the portion of the program dealing with the study of Latino culture more than those who had been here for a longer period of time. This observation needs to be tested and further interpreted, and design implications need to be considered.

RECOMMENDATIONS

It is strongly recommended that the assumptions of this program be shared through faculty briefings throughout Cuyahoga Community College and other colleges. Instructors in all subject areas need to reconsider value judgments based on less favorable views of bilingualism and to consider ways to integrate this new understanding into their work with Latino students.

Unconditional support is needed from the administration for this program to continue and succeed. Bureaucratic barriers are often in the way of innovation. The whole climate and attitude of the college personnel need to be improved. Non-motivated and non-cooperative staff members providing registration, financial aid, counseling, and information services seem to function well as effective gatekeepers. Latinos and all language/culture minority students have the right to access the existing resources and opportunities. As an urban community college, CCC must keep its gates wide open. Bilingual and bicultural staff are needed. All staff will benefit from retraining and continuing education.

Although recruitment is vital, the Horizontes experience teaches that retention is the key issue. Innovation must be encouraged and support systems are needed to respond to the special needs of the population that attends CCC. The great majority of the Latinos enrolled are female and mothers. Ethnicity and gender need to be considered while designing similar projects.

A lecture type of approach alone does not appear to be effective as a retention tool for non-traditional students. The integration of the social work with groups modality in the classroom addresses not only the awareness level but also the students' and faculty's attitudes and behavior. Faculty members recommended hiring a full-time professional social worker to teach the Latino culture class and to facilitate other student groups.

The Horizontes program design can be replicated with other cultural groups in the college. Much of what has been learned can be transferred and adapted to serve the needs of other cultural groups.

Gender is an important variable for further consideration. Much of the literature used in the Latino culture course and the topics selected aim to empower women. There is a clear feminist approach underlying the curriculum. Perhaps working-class women of different ethnic backgrounds may benefit from a Horizontes-like program as they enter college.

Social work as a profession needs to be more responsive to the needs of community-college students. Members of oppressed groups often enroll in community colleges as a first attempt to change their situation and to advance socially and economically. The community colleges of the 1990s are becoming what settlement houses were for communities in the 1950s. Social workers are needed to support these efforts and advocate for the students.

APPENDIX A

CUYAHOGA COMMUNITY COLLEGE
Project Horizontes - Latino Culture Component
Spring 1994

LIST OF READINGS

Date	Topic	Reading/Activity
01-11	Latin America	PC Globe (educational software)
01-25	Familismo	Una semana de siete días
02-01	Machismo Marianismo	Flor de Cocuyo
02-08	Fatalismo	La muñeca menor
02-15	Personalismo	Recetario de Incautos
02-22	Race and Ethnicity	Otra Maldad de Pateco
03-01	Dominicans and Peruvians	Selected readings
03-08	The Puerto Ricans	Silent Dancing
03-15	The Puerto Ricans	Silent Dancing

BIBLIOGRAPHY

Vega, José Luis (Editor). 1983. Reunión de espejos. Editorial Cultural. Rio Piedras, Puerto Rico.

- García Ramis, Magali. Una semana de siete días (pp. 111-118)
- _____. Flor de Cocuyo (pp. 119-128)
- Ferré, Rosario. La muñeca menor (pp. 145-151)
- Lugo, Filippi, Carmen. Recetario de Incautos (pp. 271-275)
- Vega, Ana Lydia. Otra Maldad de Pateco (pp. 292-300)

Oritz-Cofer, Judith. 1991. Silent Dancing: A Partial Remembrance of a Puerto Rican Childhood. Arte Publico Press: Houston.

APPENDIX B

CUYAHOGA COMMUNITY COLLEGE ● HORIZONTES - SP 243
Usando la siguiente escala, indique su opinión sobre éstas frases.

1□ 2□ 3□ 4□ 5□
muy en desacuerdo   en desacuerdo   neutral   de acuerdo   muy de acuerdo

a. Mi futuro está lleno de oportunidades.   1□ 2□ 3□ 4□ 5□
   My future is full of opportunities.

b. Obtener un bachillerato es posible para mi.   1□ 2□ 3□ 4□ 5□
   I can obtain a Bachelors degree.

c. Tengo planes de continuar mi educación.   1□ 2□ 3□ 4□ 5□
   I have plans to continue my education.

d. Problemas personales me impiden avanzar.   1□ 2□ 3□ 4□ 5□
   Personal problems don't let me advance.

e. Me siento en control de mi vida.   1□ 2□ 3□ 4□ 5□
   I feel in control of my life.

f. Me siento incómodo/a hablando inglés.   1□ 2□ 3□ 4□ 5□
   I feel uncomfortable speaking English.

g. Me siento incómodo/a en la universidad.   1□ 2□ 3□ 4□ 5□
   I feel uncomfortable at the college.

h. Me pongo nervioso/a al intervenir en clase.   1□ 2□ 3□ 4□ 5□
   I get nervous when participating in class.

i. Estando con otros hispanos me siento bien.   1□ 2□ 3□ 4□ 5□
   I feel good when I am with other Hispanics.

j. Nunca pienso en mi futuro.   1□ 2□ 3□ 4□ 5□
   I never think about my future.

k. Me siento cómodo a con los profesores.   1□ 2□ 3□ 4□ 5□
   I feel comfortable with the professors.

l. Mi familia y amigos me apoyan.   1□ 2□ 3□ 4□ 5□
   My family and friends support me.

© Marsiglia

NOTES

1. U.S. Department of Education, National Center for Education Statistics. 1993. Trends in Enrollment in Higher Education by Racial/Ethnic Category: Fall 1982 Through Fall 1991.
2. Carter, Deborah and Reginald Wilson. 1993. Minorities in Higher Education (Table 19, page 68). American Council on Education: Washington, DC.
3. U.S. Department of Education. 1992. Digest of Education Statistics, 1992. Washington, DC: National Center for Educational Statistics.

REFERENCES

Badillo-Ghali Sonia 1977. Cultural Sensitivity and the Puerto Rican Client. *Social Case Work*, 58 (8): 459-68.

Bean F. and Tienda M. 1987. *The Hispanic Population of the United States*. New York: Russell Sage Foundation.

Bird, H. R. 1982. The cultural dichotomy of colonial people. *Journal of the American Academia of Psychoanalysis,* 10:195-20.

Brinton, D.M., Snow, M.A., and Wesche, M.B. 1989. *Content-Based Second Language Instruction*. New York: Newburry House.

Cataldo, Everett F. 1990. *An Analysis of Student Outcomes for a Recent High School Cohort in the Cleveland Public Schools*. Cleveland, Ohio: Cleveland State University.

Chomsky, Noam. 1968. *The Sound Pattern of English*. New York: Harper & Row.

Clair, N. 1994. Informed choices: Articulating assumptions behind programs for language-minority students. Presentation: TESOL Convention. Baltimore: March 9, 1994. Draft.

Comas-Díaz, L. 1987. Feminist Therapy with Mainland Puerto Rican Women. *Psychology of Women Quarterly,* 11:461-474.

Flores, Juan, Attinasai, John, and Pedraza Jr., Pedro. 1981. La Carreta Made a U-Turn . . . Puerto Rican Language and Culture in the United States. *Daedalus,* 110 (2): 193-217.

Freire, Paulo. 1970. *Pedagogy of the Oppressed*. New York: Seabury.

Harding, Edith and Riley, Philip. (1986). The Bilingual Family: A Handbook for Parents. New York: Cambridge University Press.

Kuykendall, Crystal. 1992. *From Rage to Hope: Strategies for Reclaiming Black and Hispanic Students*. National Vocational Service. National Educational Services.

Kyle, Charles. 1984. Testimony to National Commission on Secondary Schooling for Hispanics. ASPIRA of Illinois.

Marsiglia, Flavio F. 1991. "Ethnic Identity and Achievement in School as Perceived by a Selected Group of Mainland Puerto Rican Students." AERA 1991 Annual Meeting: San Francisco California. ERIC Publications.

McKay, S.L. 1988. Weighing educational alternatives. In S. McKay and S.C. Wong (Eds.). *Language Diversity: Problem or Resource?* (pp. 338-366). New York: Newburry House.

Nelson C. and Tienda M. 1985. The Structuring of Hispanic Ethnicity: History and Contemporary Perspectives. *Ethnic and Racial Studies* 8:49-74.

Ovando, C.J. and Collier, V.P. 1985. *Bilingual and ESL Classrooms: Teaching in Multicultural Contexts*. New York: McGraw-Hill.

Sands, R.G. and Nuccio, K. 1992. Postmodern Feminist Theory and Social Work. *Social Work*, 37 (6):489-494.

Toseland, R.W. and Rivas, R.F. 1995. *An Introduction to Group Work Practice* (2nd edition). Boston: Allyn and Bacon.

Vygotsky, Lev. 1979. Mind in Society: *The Development of Higher Psychological Processes*. Cambridge, Mass: Harvard University Press.

Chapter 9

Group Work in Group Care

Hans G. Eriksson

A man cannot be a true father without being a creator of something, something that he wants to flourish before him rather than to have molded in his image. A true father must be an artist, otherwise he becomes a violator of the creative spirit of man, by trying to mold a child to be exactly the way he the man is . . .

Gregory Zilboorg

My frame of reference for this topic comes from two arenas of working with children and youth–as both a social worker and cottage director at a juvenile correctional institution and as a lecturer in social pedagogy about milieu treatment with children and youth at the State College of Social Work in Trondheim, Norway.

I will now allow myself to use this opportunity to share with you how my frame of reference for working with groups and group care has developed. My guiding principles, or rays of light for this journey have been lit by several people. Alan Paton's statement in *Cry, the Beloved Country*, underlining the fundamentals of human dignity–that to mean something and belong someplace is the greatest wish/need a person can have–is a dear remembrance from my first classes in social group work with Gisela Konopka. Synergy, that of bringing together the strength and resources of people in a combined effort to create a viable thrust and forceful, enriched base and quality for change and movement forward, is an influence from a

141

year spent at the School of Applied Social Science, Grace Coyle's home base at Case Western Reserve University, with Paul Abels. The importance in group work and residential work of doing things together, called activity, and the idea and reality of creating something with others I owe to Ruth Middleman. For understanding the importance of ending groups the best way, I am in debt to Helen Northen, through her ever-classical chapter on this topic, a required reading in the 1970s. In understanding, knowing, and applying developmental concepts into practice in group care, Henry Maier has lit the way for me. Thank you all very much!

The topic for this presentation is the relationship between group work and group care. We talk about residential treatment of children and youth away from their natural environment in one or another form of institutional care such as residential treatment, group care, a managed-care environment, group home, or the non-familiar living environment. "Loved child has many names," as we say in Norway. What an institution offers, for better or for worse, is a nonfamily and non-community life, and it is in these apparent negatives rather than any approximation of their positives that the value may lie. Alan Keith-Lucas (1979) outlines three major tasks that have to be carried out in regards to the child or youth entering the institution: family clarification, behavioral modification, and supplemental care.

Without having any reference point to life outside the institution, the resident will easily become a stranger both to the present place of living and where he or she came from, in addition to his or her final placement–the point being that the child/youth needs to gain some clarity in regard to which "family" is the lifeline from the outside world to the institution. This is what we in group work call reference groups, members' ties with the world outside the group, a central issue for members of a group as well as residents in institutions. The respect, liking, and wanting to belong to what one identifies as one's reference group exert power toward both negative and positive possibilities for change. Generally, the more one likes the group, the morehe or she will identify with it.

Many children and youths enter the institutional living scenario because their life space is either too full of temptation to be handled adequately, or because they do not have enough resources and flexibility to meet their needs, or possibly because they respond punitively to their activities and behavior. The children need to acquire competency, as Robert White calls it, to effectively interact with the environment. Within the institution there must be created possibilities for this, and the child care worker must be challenged "to use life events–the ordinary as well as the dramatic ones–as extraordinary opportunities to enhance the growth and development of young people in their care" (Maluccio, 1991, p. 50), and to apply these to the daily here-and-now experiences to promote each child's or youth's best interests. This is what Konopka (1983), among others, calls the purposeful choice and creation of environment through which the helping process is carried out. Individualization in group work, the recognition that the members are different and might need different attention to their particular situation, is a corollary to the concept of supplemental care. From the group care point of view this means that a particular resident might need another type or different content of care than is administered through the general program; for example, to spend the day outside the institution in a local school or place of work to expand and enrich the life space.

As noted, I parallel the use of group work and group care. There are more similarities between these two conceptual constructions than there are differences. This space is too short to make a complete comparison. As support for how the two in a synergistic way are connected to each other, I briefly point to a comment by Dave Ward (1993, p. 177), senior lecturer and head of the social work program at University of Nottingham, England, who makes the comment that day care and residential work are settings where "groups, and therefore group work, are norm [and] they should have central, not marginal, positions in the development of our theory base and repertoire of skills."

In my mind I have a picture, from my childhood on the farm, of two birch trees between which a cloth line is tied and on which several sheets, fastened with clothes pins, are blowing in the wind to get dry. Each of these sheets represent a tabula on which the principles for group work and group care are written. They have the following contents:

HUMAN DIGNITY and CARING

To mean something in the world—that is, to belong someplace where one is recognized for being—is one of the highest wants/wishes/needs we have, and is one that becomes especially important for children and youth.

We must demonstrate respect for the potential of the individual in her or his environment within the cultural context of where the person comes from and where she or he is now.

The individual must be granted autonomy to be able to live the meaning of her or his own life through caring and taking responsibility for it and not being detached from one's environment.

DEVELOPMENT

Understand behavior as "ordinary" instead of "deviant."

Focus on the reality of behavior instead of on correcting unwanted behavior.

Take small steps within a context instead of big leaps into unknown space.

Avoid forcing growth on the child or youth.

Establish interdependence between being oneself and being attached to an important other.

RELATIONSHIPS

The challenge is to achieve a togetherness; that is to strengthen the community while simultaneously enhancing the individual—an interdependence, of sorts, between the actors in the scenario.

Move away from teaching the false expectation of life. Neither the treatment group nor the residential living situation represent true life situations. They are surrogates, but as such are true in themselves and part of the total life experience of lived space and lived time.

All members are connected to other members, and members must touch each other.

USE of ACTIVITIES

Doing things (activities) together reinforces one's ability to build on already acquired skills and helps to develop new physical, cognitive, and emotional strengths.

Activities can provide unforgettable moments of exhilaration when one accomplishes new skills and breaks through new barriers.

Allow room for making a fool of oneself in a safe context.

Nature and the surrounding environment are full of easy-to-use materials.

HOPE and COURAGE

The hope for growth and development must exist. Wishful thinking or unfounded expectations are not enough. Faith and expression of the fullness of the present filled with possibilities are what is needed.

One must have the courage to challenge the unknown, based on insights and knowledge from the past, as well as trust in the others and oneself to carry out the activities needed for the situation or task.

Group work and group care have in common what we call the network of skills, knowledge, and talents that enable a person to interact with the environment. The ecological competence is composed of the person's capacities, skills, and motivation, as well as environmental qualities such as social networks, social supports, and demands or obstacles in one's ecological context. This is a shift from *treating* children and youth toward *teaching* them social skills, coping, and mastery. As Henry Maier (1991) observes in his discussion of the developmental conception of human functioning,

Life is conceived as a process in which the human being is in a continuous search for stimulation, variation, and new experience rather than a homeostatic, balanced stimuli–the existence . . . most important, a non-homeostatic conception challenges us to value people for their capacity to reach out and to develop more fully rather than for their low-risk striking for balance.

Group work and group care have also in common what Mary Follet (1918, p. 24-33) so succinctly described: that the object of a group is "to create a common idea . . . not merely to give my own ideas . . . or learn others' ideas . . . [but] . . . in order that all together we may create a group idea, an idea which will be better than all of one of our ideas alone, moreover which will be better than all of our ideas added together. For this group idea will not be produced by any process of addition, but by the interpenetration of us all." Another way of characterizing this is to use development as a metaphor, namely "as a progression of doing more with more people, doing more with more people in more places, and doing more with more people in more places at varied times" (Maier, 1991, p. 41). It is a nonlinear transformation from one stage to another of nurturing care, where the basic pattern of care is to understand the child or youth's development.

I will finish with a quote from Milton Mayeroff (1971) which for me ties group work and group care together. Here, he expounds on the intricate process of caring for others:

In caring, I experience the other as having potentialities and the need to grow; I experience an idea, for instance, as seminal, vital, or promising. In addition, I experience the other as needing me in order to grow; consider how we sometimes feel needed by another person or by a cause or an ideal. This does not simply mean that I know, in some strictly intellectual sense, that the other has needs that must be satisfied and that I can satisfy those needs. And I do not experience being needed by the other as a relationship that gives me power over it and provides me with something to dominate, but rather as a kind of trust. It is as if I had been entrusted with the care of the other in a way that is the antithesis of possessing and manipulating it as I please. (pp. 8-9)

REFERENCES

Ainsworth, F. (1987). The rush to independence . . . a new tryanny? *Australian Social Work*.

Follet, M. P. (1918). *The new state*. New York: Longmans, Green and Co.

Keith-Lucas, A. (1979). *Tasks and alternatives for the children's institution.* Chapel Hill, NC: Group Child Care Consultant Services.

Konopka, G. (1983). *Social group work: A helping process* (3rd ed.). Englewood Cliffs, NJ: Prentice-Hall.

Maier, H. W. (1987). Developmental group care of children and youth: Concepts and practice. Binghamton, NY: The Haworth Press.

Maier, H. W. (1991). Developmental foundations of child and youth care work. In J. Beker and Z. Eisikovitz (Eds.), *Knowledge utilization in residential child and youth care practice.* Washington DC: Child Welfare League of America. pp. 25-48.

Maluccio, A. N. (1991). Interpersonal and group life in residential care: A competence-centered ecological perspective. In J. Beker and Z. Eisikovits (Eds.), *Knowledge utilization in residential child and youth care practice.* Washington, DC: Child Welfare League of America. pp. 49-63.

Mayeroff, M. (1971). *On caring.* NY: Harper Collins Publishers.

Ward, Dave. (1993). *Review of Groupwork* (3rd Ed.). *Groupwork,* 6: 176-178.

Chapter 10

Group Treatment Programs for Alcoholism in the United States and Japan

Kasumi K. Hirayama
Hisashi Hirayama
Yasuhiro Kuroki

INTRODUCTION

In post-industrial societies such as the United States and Japan, alcohol abuse and alcoholism have emerged as major medical, mental health, public health, and social problems. A variety of treatment and rehabilitative programs have been developed and used by professionals in both societies. However, among the treatment approaches developed in both countries, group approaches occupy the central position in the treatment and rehabilitation of alcoholic patients.

In July 1993, we visited a well-known, model Japanese alcoholic treatment facility, Kurihama National Hospital for Alcoholism, in Kurihama, Japan. This hospital has also been designated by the World Health Organization as the main research and training center for professional staff who work with alcoholic patients in Japan. We spent a day observing the program and talked with the director of the hospital and his staff on their views of Japanese alcohol problems and the alcohol treatment program at the hospital. One of us has also had experience working at a substance abuse residential treatment facility in Connecticut in 1994, and has visited other substance abuse treatment facilities in that state. Based on field studies and a review of American and Japanese literature on alco-

149

holism, this paper compares and contrasts major group treatment programs currently being used in residential facilities for alcoholism in the United States and Japan. Specific attention is given to similarities and differences in American and Japanese attitudes toward drinking, treatment goals, group treatment components, group practice models and structures, and treatment outcomes.

Alcohol dependence and alcoholism are serious problems that affect about 10 percent of adult Americans (DHHS, 1990, p. xxi). An estimated 10.5 million U.S. adults exhibit some symptoms of alcoholism or alcohol dependence, and an additional 7.2 million abuse alcohol but do not yet show symptoms of dependence (DHHS, 1990, p. ix). Kinney and Laton (1991) report that approximately 72 percent of the adult U.S. population drinks, including 77 percent of men and 67 percent of women. An estimate of one out of five adolescents aged 14 to 17 have drinking problems, totaling 2.8 million teenagers. Nationwide concern about alcohol use among adolescents has led to mandated school-based drug and alcohol education programs in every state; yet a study by the University of Michigan Institute for Social Research on secondary school and college students' drinking found that while it was illegal for all high school students and most college students to purchase alcohol, 88 percent of high school seniors have tried alcohol (Johnson, O'Malley, and Buchman, 1992, pp. 12-18). Thirty percent of high school seniors in the study reported that most or all of their friends got drunk once a week. In terms of availability, 67 percent of eighth graders and 84 percent of tenth graders reported that they could obtain alcohol fairly easily (pp. 195-196). These data clearly indicate that alcohol abuse and/or alcohol dependence is very prevalent among the U.S. population.

In Japan, close to 90 percent of the adult population drinks alcohol; 50 percent of adult males and 10 percent of adult females drink daily. An estimated 3.6 percent of the adult population exhibits symptoms of alcohol dependence (Kono, 1992, p. 150). Along with the remarkable economic growth and development in Japan, alcohol consumption has shown a steady increase in the past 30 years, particularly among young people, including high school students and women. In 1979, alcohol consumption was six times greater than pre-World War II era consumption. A survey conducted by Koseisho (the Ministry of Health and Welfare) showed an estimate of 2,220,000 alcoholics in Japan in 1985 (Ichimura, 1986, p. 144). Social drinking, which used to be limited to men, has become popular among women and young people, including teens. Attractively designed beer cans; sweet wine mixed with fruit juices; 200,000 beer, wine, and liquor vending machines located all over Japan (Kono, 1992, p. 110); and daily repetitious TV commercials for beer, wine, and liquor have rendered the habitual use of alcohol among the Japanese very prevalent. Societal prevention of alcohol abuse has been minimal. Since 1921, there has been a Japanese law forbidding young people, 20 years of age and under, from drinking; however, there have been no laws to deal with young people's drinking. Therefore, no arrests can be made if teens are caught drinking.

According to one nationwide survey of 15,222 high school students, about 60 percent of them drink; one out of four boys and one out of ten girls were designated as "problem drinkers," who consume three to six glasses of beer or wine in a one-week period (Kono, 1992, p. 150).

AMERICAN AND JAPANESE
CULTURAL CONTEXTS

Although American and Japanese treatment programs resemble each other on the surface, because of the contextual differences in their respective cultures, such as attitudinal differences on drinking and degrees of gender bias associated with drinking, treatment programs, as well as the structure and content of the programs, differ in these societies.

The United States has gone through several changes in attitudes and practices involving alcohol. *Colonial views* on alcohol were not restrictive. Alcohol was widely available and drinking was generally tolerated. Although drunkenness was commonplace, it was not considered a social problem until the nation became an urban industrial economy instead of an agrarian economy in the early 1700s to the mid-1800s (Jung, 1994, p. 6). This era saw the heaviest alcohol consumption in American history (Robertson, 1988, p. 43). The widespread social problems created by use of alcohol raised the public awareness, leading to the Temperance Movement in 1833 to eliminate alcohol. The movement was strongly influenced by Protestant Christians and eventually led to the passage of the Volstead Act in 1919, legally abolishing alcohol consumption. During the Temperance and Prohibition Eras, drinking was judged immoral. Excessive drinking was deemed a sinful behavior stemming from character defects and reflecting a lack of willpower. "Little sympathy was given to the drunkard, who was ridiculed as a skid-row bum" (Jung, 1994, p. 7; DHHS, 1990, p. 3). The Prohibition Era did not last long as illegal alcohol was widely available, and the Act was repealed in 1932 (Jung, 1994). For years, alcoholics have labeled themselves wicked, weak, and reprehensible (Vaillant, 1983, p. 19), reflecting lingering societal moral views on alcoholics from the Prohibition Era.

In the United States, Alcoholics Anonymous, a self-help program initiated by two alcoholics in 1935, led to a major shift in society's attitude toward alcoholism, moving away from the moral model to the disease model. Scientific examination of alcoholism also began in the 1930s.

Today, excessive drinking is viewed in the United States as demonstrating impaired control in limiting alcohol intake; alcohol dependence is viewed as the end result of an "interactive process involving many different social and psychological factors in persons who are physiologically vulnerable" (Tarter et al., 1985; DHHS, 1990, p. 6).

The Japanese attitudes and behaviors toward alcohol have historically been very tolerant. Japanese religions, especially Shintoism, have played a significant role in shaping Japanese attitudes toward alcohol. Early Shintoism, which goes back more than 2,000 years, centered around the animistic worship of natural phenomenon–the sun, mountains, trees, water, etc.–and the whole process of fertility. No line was drawn between man and nature (Reischauer, 1977). Thus, Japanese wine, *sake*, made from rice harvested in the fall, has been used in the rituals of Shinto religion. Deities have been worshipped through offerings such as sake, harvested crops, food, flowers, prayers, and lighthearted, jovial festivals at shrines. Heavy drinking among men at festival times is commonplace. Alcohol has been used for men as the rite of passage into adulthood from adolescence. Americans also use alcohol ceremonially in Holy Communion in churches and in wedding and other toasts. Some use it as a rite of passage, along with losing one's virginity.

Japanese ceremonial use of alcohol has extended to weddings, funerals, business entertainments, and all kinds of parties. Japanese weddings at Shinto shrines use Japanese wine for ceremony and Western wines for the wedding luncheon or dinner after the ceremony. On funeral occasions, families of the deceased serve mourners sake and food during the wake and after the funeral.

Alcohol has been used extensively by businessmen for entertaining their counterparts in business dealings. This has been further extended to all sorts of parties held by business firms for their employees. It is customary to accept wine when offered by one's superior at these parties. Japanese men are allowed to become drunk and be very expressive at such parties–the only time such behavior is allowed in the nonverbally oriented Japanese culture. Showing talents such as individual singing, dancing, and group singing are common behaviors at parties.

The Japanese attitude toward women's drinking, however, has been more restrictive than that toward men's. Excessive drinking by women has been viewed by the public as vulgar and indecent. Women, therefore, are excused for not drinking. As increasing numbers of Japanese women have entered the business and professional fields, and as present Japanese law forbids differential treatment of women, there has been a shift from the negative view of women's drinking to more positive views, espoused by liberated women and outgoing women. The rule for women's drinking is not to become drunk in public.

Excessive drinking by men at New Year's parties, festivals, and many other business-related and family parties is tolerated, but the cardinal rule is not to drive a car when drinking. If a person is caught driving while intoxicated or has an accident caused by drunken driving, his situation will change dramatically. His driver's license may be revoked, depending on the severity and frequency of incidents. Once a person's occupation, such as teacher or government official, appears in the newspaper, his job may be in jeopardy. There is also the social stigma of treatment for alcoholism.

Thus, the Japanese societal attitude toward drinking is very contradictory. On one hand, drinking is encouraged and is used heavily; on the other hand, once a Japanese adult crosses the line of decency or adequate control, he is judged to be morally weak with character defects. He may be ostracized by society and distanced from his intimate circle.

GROUP TREATMENT PROGRAMS
IN THE UNITED STATES AND JAPAN

Treatment Philosophy and Goals for Alcoholism

Many treatment programs for alcoholism in the United States adhere to the Minnesota model of rehabilitation (Johnson, 1980; Institute of Medicine, 1990; Jung, 1994). This is conceptualized in a three-stage recovery model: (1) detoxification for up to a week, (2) rehabilitation (residential and/or day treatment) for 14 to 28 days (becoming shorter every year by changes in insurance coverage, and (3) aftercare (Alterman, O'Brien, and McLellan, 1991).

The treatment philosophy is that chemical dependence is a disease, not a mental disorder or a failure of morals, intellect, or will-power, as once believed. Admitting one's dependence is the first step in the healing process of recovery for addicted men and women, as well as their families.

Based on this philosophy, the major goals of treatment in the residential program are learning to overcome denial, learning to cope with obstacles to abstinence, and medical stabilization, if necessary (Alterman, O'Brien, and McLellan, 1991, p. 372). Abstinence for life is the ultimate goal of treatment.

In comparison with the American treatment program, the Japanese treatment program is longer, at least three months, and can be extended to six months due to the liberal national health insurance coverage, which pays the total cost of treatment. Because of the extreme societal tolerance of drinking, many addicted Japanese enter the treatment facility in worse physical conditions than their American counterparts, with cirrhosis of the liver, stomach ulcer, kidney disease, malnutrition, and mental dementia. Because of social stigma, the majority of addiction problems are treated in general hospitals under the disguise of other physical illnesses. Only extreme cases are treated at specialized hospitals such as Kurihama Hospital. Therefore, specialized facilities to treat alcoholism are still limited. By 1986, there were two hospitals for alcoholism, six hospitals with alcoholic units, seven public health clinics, and two youth development centers that devoted their services to alcohol-related problems (Ichimura, 1986, p. 145).

The Kurihama treatment philosophy (see Table 10.1) is that alcohol is a major risk factor leading to serious diseases. If one chooses to drink, it is his or her freedom to decide, but one has to pay the price. If one cannot control his or her drinking, he or she has to be sober for life. Alcohol dependence, in this sense, is still viewed as a failure of self-control. One can be helped to sobriety through joint responsibility among patients for learning about alcoholism and healing oneself, based on a horizontal clinician-patient team approach in an open system, rather than the traditional hierarchical medical model (Kono, 1992). Alcoholism is not clearly defined as a disease.

Based on the above philosophy, the major treatment goals for alcoholism are (1) to become sober through studying and working together; (2) to establish an orderly, routine life; and (3) to return to normal social functioning in one's own community. Abstinence for life is not clearly stated to be the ultimate treatment goal.

TABLE 10.1. Treatment Philosophy and Goals

United States	*Japan*
Philosophy: Chemical dependence is *a disease*, not a mental disorder or a failure of morals, intellect, or willpower. Admitting one's dependence is the first step in the healing process of recovery for addicted men and women, as well as their families.	**Philosophy:** Alcohol is *a major risk factor* leading to serious diseases. If one cannot control his or her drinking, he or she has to be sober for life.
Goals: Learning to overcome denial and learning to cope with obstacles to abstinence	**Goals:** Learning to become sober through studying and working together, and returning to normal social functioning in his or her community
Ultimate Goal (stated): Abstinence for life	**Ultimate Goal (implied):** Abstinence for life

Group Treatment Components

Group treatment is the primary method in treating alcoholism in both American and Japanese programs. An American treatment program consists of a number of components:

1. Daily *group therapy* focuses on individual experiences and feelings associated with chemical dependency and is conducted like a clinician-patient one-on-one session within a group.
2. *Education sessions* are a mixture of didactic films and lectures about the physical, mental, and psychological effects of alcohol.
3. *Journal* consists of daily, individual journal writing on the patient's thoughts and feelings, which are read in a group meeting.
4. *Nutrition and medical treatment* are tailored to individual needs.
5. *Participation in A.A./N.A.* or other self-help group meetings is a part of most residential treatment programs or a post-treatment supplement.
6. *Creative therapy* includes art, movement, and/or occupational therapy.
7. *Community meetings,* including staff members, are held daily at the end of the treatment sessions at many centers to evaluate the day's activities and events as a group.
8. *Individual and family counseling* is conducted at least twice–at the time of admission and before discharge. Except in components (4) and (8), the group is the primary method of providing these program components. In other words, about 90 percent of the treatment program uses groups as a primary treatment method.

The Japanese treatment program, during the rehabilitative period after detoxification, includes an even broader array of components.

1. *Physical exercise* is scheduled every morning for ten minutes using a radio physical exercise program.
2. *Weekly medical check-ups and treatment* are provided on the basis of need.
3. *Five-minute meditations* are held twice a day, after the physical exercise session and after dinner.

4. At the *self-study group,* the patients use many available resources to study alcoholism among themselves, without professional assistance.

5. An *education group* is held once a week for one and one-half hours, at which the staff lectures on alcohol dependence.

6. Attendance at a monthly *abstinence self-help group,* where 30-minute reports are given by members on their abstinence activities is required. A.A. reports on its activities (which are different from the abstinence self-help group) biweekly.

7. *Group therapy*/small group meetings focus on patients' experiences and feelings associated with alcohol dependence. There are all kinds of small group meetings—unit group meetings, subgroup meetings, group leaders' meetings, bimonthly group meeting with a social worker, monthly meetings with graduates (former patients), nursing meetings, orientation group meeting, before home-visit/after home-visit group meeting, discharge group meetings, etc.

8. *Work/occupational therapy* aims to regain the patients' physical functioning through gardening in the flower and vegetable gardens. Some other activities include a patients' newsletter group, which collects newspaper articles on alcohol-related issues and makes scrapbooks. Newspaper articles are not limited to Japanese. Some are world news on addiction from English newspapers.

9. *Art therapy* is used as an assessment tool as well as a way for patients to develop and express their creativity through painting and craft activities. Final projects are exhibited in an art show and decorate the treatment facility inside and out.

10. *Recreation therapy* is designed to help patients become cooperative and enjoy each other through games.

11. *Walking* as therapy takes two forms—walking as a group several miles once a week and taking a walk around the grounds alone. Group walking emphasizes sweating and suffering together to face physical hardship and share the same experience in order to solidify as a group. Walking alone is for meditative and introspective purposes.

12. *Cleaning* is assigned to a small group, and each group is assigned to certain tasks of cleaning in order to develop routine habits of making a clean, pleasant environment.
13. *Evaluation/reflection time* is held every evening after brief meditation. This is similar to a community meeting at treatment centers in the United States to evaluate the day's activities and events. Patients can ask questions on unclear matters and discuss issues of their concern at this time.
14. *Family meetings* are held bi-monthly.
15. *Home visit*, the third month of stay, is the patients' transition period from hospitalization back to the community. Home visits are scheduled and group meetings before home visits and after home visits are held. Patients are also strongly encouraged to belong to self-help groups of their choice (Abstinence group or Alcoholics Anonymous).

Almost 95 percent of the Japanese treatment components are conducted in groups. There are more group activities in the Japanese program, such as daily physical exercise, daily group cleaning weekly long-distance group walking, a newsletter group, flower and vegetable gardening, before and after discharge groups, and many other group meetings with a social worker, nurses, former patients, etc.

Components such as group therapy, education group, art, recreation, occupational therapies (work group), and community meeting, or evaluation/reflection time as a group, are very similar in both programs. (See Table 10.2.) However, their group practice model and group structure are different in the United States and Japan. (See Table 10.3.)

Group Practice Model and Group Structure

Groups in the treatment programs for alcoholism in the United States, viewed from a social group work perspective, are conducted strictly in the clinical model. Goals and purposes are clearly stated. The clinician-patient relationship is inclined to be up-to-down with clinicians as experts. The social worker's role is that of change agent. Most of the rules and regulations are made by the professional staff, and patients participate minimally in the decision-making process.

TABLE 10.2. Components of Inpatient Treatment Programs for Alcoholism

United States	*Japan*
Daily affirmation (ind.): 15 min.	Physical exercise (gr.), daily: 10 min.
Group therapy, daily: 1 & 1/2 hrs.	Meditation (ind.), 2/daily: 5 min. each.
Movement therapy (gr.), 2/wk.: 1 hr.	Work group (small gr.), 2/wk.: 30 min.
Cleanup (ind.), 2/wk.: 1 hr.	Study group, 2/wk.: 30 min.
Education (gr.), daily: 1 hr.	Group therapy - open, 1/wk.: 1 hr.
Journal writing (ind.)	Group therapy - closed, 1/wk.: 1 hr.
Journal reading (gr.), daily: 30 min.	Arts and crafts (gr.), 1/wk.
Reading (ind.), 2/wk.: 1 hr.	Art therapy, (ind.), 1/wk.
Aerobics (gr.), 2/wk.: 1 hr.	Stress management (gr.), 1/wk.
Art therapy (gr.), 2/wk.: 1 hr.	Medical checkup (ind.), 1/wk.
Medical checkup (ind.)	Music therapy (gr.), 1/wk.: 1 hr.
Community meeting (gr.), daily: 30 min.*	Education (gr.), 1/wk.: 1 hr.
AA/NA meetings (gr.), 2/wk.	Walking (gr.), 1/wk.: 3-5 miles.
Individual and family meetings, at the admission and before discharge.	Walking (ind.), daily: grounds.
	Reports on Abstinence or AA (gr.), 2/mon.
	Group meeting w/ social worker, bi-monthly.
	Group meeting w/ graduates, monthly.
	Before home visit/after home visit (gr.).
	Other groups (unit meeting, discharge group, newsletter group, family meeting, etc.).

*Some programs do not have community meetings.

TABLE 10.3. Group Practice Model and Group Structure

United States	Japan
Practice model: Clinical	Practice model: Interactional
Open-ended, short-term group, 14 to 28 days	Open-ended, long-term group, 90 to 180 day.
Structure: Dyads or togetherness w/less group cohesion and less use of group process	Structure: Elected leaders w/observable structure and cohesion, and good use of group process

As the U.S. treatment programs are short and open-ended, with some patients entering and some leaving weekly, there is not much time to develop a clear group structure with indigenous leaders and subgroup members in a pecking order. Also, the creation of such a group may not be encouraged by clinicians. Structure is given and enforced by the treatment staff to patients. Use of the group process in the treatment group sessions by clinicians are limited, and it tends to be more individual dialogue between the patient and the clinician in a group while group members are asked to listen.

In comparison with U.S. programs, Japanese treatment programs for alcoholism use group processes fully. Although the outlook of the program is in a medical model with specific behavioral change to remedy dysfunction, the core of the treatment program is conducted in the interactional model. Clinicians' roles are more those of resource people. The approach is more humanitarian than autocratic. Program components are designed to create a cohesive atmosphere conducive to cooperation. Whereas American programs tend to be more verbally oriented, Japanese programs are nonverbally oriented. Patients in the Japanese program are organized into small groups with leaders who are elected by the group members. Although the treatment schedule is planned by clinicians, the implementation of the schedule is done by the patient group. Leaders use group pressure to enforce rules and regulations decided upon by clinicians and patients together. The length of Japanese treatment groups helps to solidify the patients' group structure. The mutual help and cooperation among patients, sharing hard work and happiness together, the use of small groups to accomplish chores in routine daily activities, and the full use of group process are the primary vehicles for accomplishing treatment goals.

SUMMARY

Although inpatient treatment programs in both countries utilize groups as the primary method of treatment they do so very differently. The Japanese program emphasizes cultivation of a sense of cooperation, sharing, and group solidarity through many kinds of patient activity-oriented groups, which are run mostly by patient leaders. In comparison, emphasis is placed on the development of self-identity, self-esteem, and individual achievement in American programs. The Japanese sense of self-identity is enmeshed with the group they belong to, unlike Americans.

Treatment programs in the United States are very verbally oriented, whereas programs in Japan are not. The Japanese use nonverbal stress management activities combined with activities for behavioral self-control.

The goal of American treatment is succinctly stated as abstinence for life, whereas the Japanese put it less forcefully, although abstinence for life is their ultimate goal.

As Japanese societal tolerance for alcohol intoxication is high, Japanese alcoholics come to the hospital in worse condition than their American counterparts. The success rate of treatment in Japan, if defined as abstinence from alcohol for two years after discharge, is 20 to 30 percent, according to Dr. Kono (1993).

The success rate of treatment with American programs varies widely from 50 percent or above to 7 percent (Jung, 1994, p. 203). Nathan (1986) reports that some evaluations by private institutions on middle and upper middle-class alcoholics showed one-year abstinence rates on the order of 50 percent and above; while one-year abstinence rates with "poorly motivated, older, single, unemployed chronic alcoholics" are 25 percent or lower (Nathan, 1986; Alterman, O'Brien, and McLellan, 1991, p. 372). And according to Emrick and Hansen (1983), the Rand study with random samplings of 474 patients over 4.5 years showed a 7 percent success rate (Jung, 1994, p. 203). Further research is needed in the area of treatment effectiveness as there is a scarcity of research on the effectiveness of each treatment component. Treatment programs reflect their cultural contexts. The definition of alcoholism differs between the United States and Japan, with the latter's criterion more loose than the American. No specific treatment program will work for all alcoholics. However, there may be room for improvement in programs in the United States and Japan alike by accepting different techniques for which evidence of effectiveness exists.

BIBLIOGRAPHY

Alterman, A.I., O'Brien, C.P., and McLellan, A.T. (1991). Differential therapeutics for substance abuse. In Frances, R.J. and Miller, S.I. (Eds.), *Clinical Textbook of Addictive Disorders*. New York: The Guilford Press.

Emrick, C.D., and Hansen, J. (1983). Assertions regarding effectiveness of treatment for alcoholism: Fact or fantasy? *American Psychologist*, 38: 1078-1088.

Ichimura, K. (1986). Alcohol related problems and the role of the treatment facility for alcoholism, *Osaka Social Welfare Study, Number 9,* December: 143-151.

Institute of Medicine (1990). *Broadening the Base of Treatment for Alcohol Problems*. Washington, DC: National Academy Press.

Jellinek, E.M. (1960). *The Disease Concept of Alcoholism*. New Haven, CT: Hill House.

Johnson, V.E. (1980). *I'll Quit Tomorrow*. San Francisco, CA: Harper & Row.

Johnson, L.O., O'Malley, P.M., and Buchman, L.G. (1992). Smoking, drinking and illicit drug use among American secondary school students, college students, and young adults, 1975-1991. *Secondary School Students*. Washington, DC: U.S. Government Printing Office.

Jung, J. (1994). *Under the Influence: Alcohol and Human Behavior*. Pacific Grove, CA: Brooks/Cole Publishing.

Kinney, J. and Leaton, G. (1991). *Loosening the Grip: A Handbook of Alcohol Information*. St. Louis, MO: Mosby Year Book.

Kono, H. (1992). *From Kurihama Alcohol Unit: Wisdom of 30 Years of Clinical Practice*. Tokyo: Toho-Shobo Publishing.

Kono, H. (July 1993). Interview with Dr. Kono.

Nathan, P.E. (1986). Treatment outcomes for alcoholism in the U.S.; Current research. In Lorberg, T., Miller, W.R., Nathan, P.E. and G.A. Marlatt (Eds.), *Addictive Behaviors: Prevention and Early Intervention*. Amsterdam: Swets & Zeitlinger. 87-101.

Reischauer, E. (1977). *The Japanese*. Cambridge, MA: The Belknap Press.

Robertson, N. (1988). *Getting Better: Inside Alcoholics Anonymous*. New York: Fawcett Press.

Tartar, R.E., Alterman, A.I., and Edwards, K.L. (1985). Vulnerability to alcoholism in men: A behavior-genetic perspective. *J. Stud Alcohol*, 46(4): 329-356.

U.S. DHHS (January, 1990). *Seventh Special Report to the U.S. Congress on Alcohol and Health.* Washington, DC: Government Printing Office (ADM), 90-1656.

Vaillant, G.E. (1983). *The Natural History of Alcoholism.* Cambridge, MA: Harvard University Press.

Chapter 11

Distance Education
and Social Group Work:
The Promise of the Year 2000

John J. Conklin
Warren Osterndorf

INTRODUCTION

Social work practice today is faced with a startling array of
dilemmas. Social problems are increasing at an astounding rate if
judged by the frequency with which the daily newspapers report the
incidence of gang crimes, poverty, homelessness, drug abuse, rapes,
robberies, family violence, and a variety of other community issues.

Social work education and practice has been forced to confront a
series of equally perplexing dilemmas. Stated simply, *we are being
required to expand the accessibility and quality of social work
services during a time when the financial resources for higher
education and social agencies are shrinking rapidly.*

A partial answer to these dilemmas is that both schools of social
work and social agencies need to consider using distance education as
a vehicle that can deliver more education and training to more students
and social work practitioners more quickly at any geographic distance.
The effectiveness and cost savings will be described.

A recent *U.S– News and World Report* (March 21, 1994) article
reported that the number of students receiving master's degrees in
social work has jumped by 31 percent since 1988. This is attributed to
the interest in what was termed "America's No. 1 Problem: Gang
Violence." Related social work issues were noted to be spousal abuse

and other "urban ills." Traditionally, these issues have been within the province of social group workers within the profession (Alissi, 1980).

In addition to the obvious need for services to inner-city youth and schools, family systems, in general, are in need of comprehensive approaches as more children are being raised in single-parent families. Levine and Associates (1990) make demographic projections that will also have an impact upon social work services. As noted by these studies, the population of this country is aging. This portends the need for more social workers to provide health care services to the elderly.

Both ends of the spectrum point to the need for additional trained social workers. How many? One projection offered by the Bureau of Labor Statistics (1992) is that at least 20,000 more social workers per year will be needed for the next 15 years to meet anticipated societal problems.

An answer to how these social workers will be located and trained can be linked to the rapid development of technology and the Internet. One of the newest types of technology uses interactive television called "distance education" or "distance learning" for training, staff development, continuing education, and the rapid transmission of information to any geographic site.

This chapter provides a definition of distance education and a description of several applications. It also spells out how distance education can be used for social group work education, field education, and social group work practice in a variety of community settings.

DEFINITION OF DISTANCE EDUCATION

The Office of Technology Assessment of the United States Congress (1989) defines distance education as: "the linking of a teacher and students in several geographic locations via technology that allows for interaction." This definition identifies both the teacher and the learner as being part of the same instructional event. Second, the teacher and the learner are separated by some geographical distance. Third, they are linked by technology that allows them to interact, no matter what the distance is.

The actual use of distance education is growing at both the undergraduate and graduate levels of higher education. In 1985, over

100,000 college students were enrolled in credit courses delivered in a distance learning environment in the United States (Brock, 1985). Meanwhile, in business, over 40 percent of the Fortune 500 companies used distance learning to deliver worksite education (Moore et al., 1990).

Collaborative ventures such as the National Technological University (NTU) have also been formed between businesses and universities to deliver education to the worksite. Distance education has enabled students to complete entire graduate degrees at the worksite. This approach has eliminated costly travel to distant campuses.

TYPES OF DISTANCE EDUCATION

A basic interactive distance learning system involves one-way video and two-way audio reception. In this system, students at several remote sites see and hear the instructor who transmits from a technology-equipped classroom. This includes several video cameras connected to a computer that sends a signal via satellite, telephone line, or point-to-point microwave transmission.

Students can communicate with the instructor by using an interactive telephone link. In this case, the instructor does not see the students but can talk directly with them at several geographic sites.

Several other variations of one-way video, two-way audio distance learning systems are available. These are delivered by satellite, cable television, or a closed-circuit system. In these systems, the audio and video portion of the program are delivered by satellite while the students' responses to the instructor are carried by ordinary telephone lines.

The more sophisticated distance learning systems use two-way video and two-way audio transmission facilities. In these systems, the instructor can see, hear, and interact with students who, in turn, can see, hear, and interact with the instructor. Often called "two-way" or "fully interactive systems," this technology projects both audio and video signals so that both students and instructors can participate in a dialog from several sites. Several television sets at each site connect all of the classrooms together.

Another type of fully interactive system is called an "interactive compressed video system" (ICV). Students and instructors who use this technology are again fully interactive as far as audio and video signals are concerned. What is different is that a complicated technology called "compression-decompression" known as "Codec" actually compresses the video signal so that it can be sent over telephone lines. On the other end, the signal is "decompressed" and shown on television sets on the other end. Interaction between the students and instructors are again spontaneous.

Costs for the various systems vary quite a bit. However, a large number of newer systems are being developed in the business community. The result is that costs are coming down rapidly, and the technology is increasing greatly in quality. Distance education is rapidly becoming "affordable."

DISTANCE EDUCATION
AND SOCIAL GROUP WORK TRAINING

How could social group work agencies and schools of social work use distance education? For workers or students who live some geographic distance away from the agency or school, conferences and classes about group work techniques can be sent to local sites. For schools, this includes courses at the undergraduate, graduate, and doctoral levels since virtually all can be transmitted via interactive television.

In addition, "live" observations of groups in process can be sent back to schools from transmission sites such as hospitals and public broadcasting facilities that are already equipped for distance education. There, classes can observe groups in action, record the transmission on videotape, and analyze group processes through using techniques such as SYMLOG (Kutner and Kirsch, 1985).

Continuing education classes may be transmitted for new field instructors who need to be taught how to supervise students who work with groups. Also, many practitioners needing continuing education credits who live some distance from the school of social work can take a variety of undergraduate and graduate courses via distance learning technology.

Earlier, distance education was used for those who were considered to be "geographically disadvantaged." At the present, "distance" is no longer synonymous with "rural" (Raymond, 1988) since the technology can be used in large metropolitan areas where "cross-town" travel is slow. This has been done over the past decade for urban hospital teaching by medical and nursing schools (Kuramoto, 1984).

Much of social work education is still being presented through the blackboard and discussion format in the classroom with concurrent field education in social agencies. Traditionally, students have driven to the school and to their agency placements for education. Today's adult learners are having increasing difficulty balancing their part-time educational schedules with full-time employment, day care, transportation, and time lost away from home, school, and their workplace.

Travel and travel time have become even more expensive propositions since most regular classes are still taught "at school." Conferences with the faculty advisor are held "at school." The seminar for field instructors is taught "at school." Finally, consultants from the schools have to travel throughout a large area to visit each student "at the agency." These practices can now be modified toward greater cost-effectiveness since all of the above can be done through distance education technology. Greater cost effectiveness can be experienced just through savings in travel and time costs. The American business community has already learned this lesson (Conklin, 1993).

OTHER APPLICATIONS FOR SOCIAL WORK SCHOOLS AND AGENCIES

Other services can be developed through distance education. Busy agency executives usually have difficulty breaking away from tight schedules to travel to planning committees or board meetings at schools of social work. National lecturers and scholars often find it difficult to travel to schools to make their presentations. Schools are finding that the cost of travel to bring a national authority to their campus has become evermore prohibitive.

Presently, to convene a panel of social work experts who travel any distance is extremely expensive. To assemble an interdisciplinary panel of experts from several fields is both difficult to coordinate as well as to afford. How cost effective would it be if panelists were asked to make a distance education presentation at their home university via telephone line, rather than to fly across the nation to participate?

NEW COURSES FOR NEW MARKETS

Not only can the required social group work courses be taught to students through distance education, there are many that could be offered to other professionals. Social work is not the only profession today that is concerned with family systems, groups, civil rights, domestic violence, care for people with AIDS and HIV, substance abuse, urban violence, gangs, relationship therapy, and brief treatment. Courses taught by social work faculty can now be transmitted to reception sites at other universities, colleges, community colleges, and professional schools throughout the nation with the technology that is available. The requisite fees would be paid to the university that taught the course. This would be a new "market" for schools of social work and agencies.

Ultimately, as costs go down, faculty members will profit from conferences with some of their distinguished colleagues in the country via satellite or telephone transmission on any number of topics. American business already uses this format nationally and internationally.

Many affordable programs are already available through the Public Broadcasting System Adult Learning Satellite Service. They include the pioneering work community colleges and others have done already on distance education for undergraduate students (Connecticut Distance Learning Consortium live video conference, Hartford, March 23, 1994).

FIELD EDUCATION

The above includes the teaching carried on outside the school known as Field Education. Several technologies can be used here. Through field education units (Conklin and Borecki, 1991) or learning laboratories, students, agency personnel, school faculty, and field faculty can have supervisory conferences via e-mail or a distance learning format. A cost-benefit analysis of the travel, time, and associated expenses would prove interesting compared to the cost of electronic transmission of the conference.

This leads directly to using the distance education potential of the "information superhighway" known as Internet. Through this large computer network, students, agencies, and schools of social work can exchange information, do library searches, and establish a variety of databases. In fact, social workers can now communicate with each other throughout the world about common issues.

QUESTIONS FOR FURTHER DISCUSSION

An interesting instructional question related to distance education, social group work education, and agency practice is developing: "*If many schools of social work and social agencies may eventually communicate across local, regional, and national boundaries, what effects will this have on the profession?*" Associated questions include whether this will improve practice, change practice, have no impact whatsoever, or have a deleterious effect. When group work takes on a more international mission, will new models, new theories, and new research need to be initiated? Or, do we already have quite enough to use in the world crises that appear on every front page every day?

An optimistic answer to this is that distance education can only serve to strengthen social group work. Soon, students will "take classes" with some of the greatest educators in the country. National committees and colleagues can "meet" without having to travel thousands of miles to do it. The national conference may be presented using evermore distance education to reach throughout the country and perhaps the world in a few years. Group work colleagues will communicate more rapidly and more thoroughly between schools and agencies interactively as they describe their newest approaches for gang violence, the prevention of family breakdown, family therapy, community mental health, and similar emerging topics. All of these issues will continue to be at the forefront of practice in the next several years before the year 2000.

SOLUTIONS

Another type of proactive approach regarding the uses of technology and distance education concerns starting a large strategic planning process based upon data that are already available (Conklin, 1993). Using some of the principles initiated by Deming (Brandt, 1992) in his "total quality management" paradigm, social group workers can position themselves to meet the opportunities promised by technology for the millennium.

It has long been a part of the "commitments and perspectives" (Alissi, 1980) of social group work to engage in active community planning so as to foster democratic change. There are now some growing challenges and opportunities to use distance education, technology-enhanced practice, and the latest advancements to facilitate and enrich the basic mission of social group work.

BIBLIOGRAPHY

Alissi, A. (1980). *Perspectives on social group work practice: A book of readings.* New York: Free Press.

Brandt, R. (1992). On Deming and school quality: A conversation with Enid Brown. *Educational Leadership,* 50: 28-31.

Brock, D. (1985). PBS tunes into adult learning. In E. E. Miller and M. L. Moseley (Eds.), *Educational Media and Technology Yearbook, Vol. II.* Littleton, CO: Libraries Unlimited, 49-53.

Conklin, J. J. (1993). The development of strategic plans for implementing distance education in social work education. Fort Lauderdale: Nova University Programs for Higher Education (ERIC Document Reproduction Service No. ED 360 892).

Conklin, J. J. and Borecki, M. C. (1991). Field education units revisited: A model for the 1990's. In D. Schneck, B. Grossman, and U. Glassman (Eds.), *Field Education in Social Work: Contemporary Issues and Trends.* Dubuque, IA: Kendall/Hunt.

Falk, D. R. and Carlson, H. L. (1992). Learning to teach with multimedia. *Technological Horizons in Education,* 20: 96-101.

Kuramoto, A. (1984). Teleconferencing for nurses: Evaluating its effectiveness. In L. Parker and C. Olgren (Eds.), *Teleconferencing and Electronic Communications III.* Madison, WI: University of Wisconsin Extension.

Kutner, S. S. and Kirsch, R. D. (1985). Clinical applications of SYMLOG: A graphic system of observing relationships. *Social Work,* 6: 497-503.

Levine, A. and Associates. (1990). *Shaping Higher Education's Future: Demographic Realities and Opportunities, 1990-2000.* San Francisco, CA: Jossey-Bass.

Moore, M. G., Thompson, M. M., Quigley, B. A., Clark, G. C., and Goff, G. G. (1990). The effects of distance learning: A summary of literature, monograph number 2. University Park, PA: The American Center for the Study of Distance Education.

Raymond, F. B. (1988). Providing social work education and training in rural areas through interactive television. (ERIC Document Reproduction Service No. ED 309 910).

Shapiro, J. J. and Hughes, S. K. (1992). Networked information resources in distance graduate education for adults. *Technological Horizons in Education*, 19: 66-69.

U.S. Congress, Office of Technology Assessment. (1989) *Linking for Learning: A New Course for Education*, OTA-SET-430. Washington, DC: U.S. Government Printing Office.

U.S. Department of Labor, Bureau of Labor Statistics, (Spring 1992). "The 1990-2005 Job Outlook in Brief," *Occupational Outlook Quarterly.*

U.S. News and World Report (March 21, 1994). Social work and public health: Tackling violence on city streets–and the campus–students and faculty grapple with America's no. 1 problem, 116: 11.

Verduin, J. R. and Clark, T. A. (1991). *Distance Education.* San Francisco, CA: Jossey-Bass.

Index

Page numbers followed by the letter "t" indicate a table.

T - #0245 - 101024 - C0 - 212/152/11 [13] - CB - 9780789001382 - Gloss Lamination